I0875876

AI for Biomedical Research Volume 1 From Idea to Analysis

Artificial intelligence (AI) is transforming every aspect of biomedical research practice. Researchers face a fragmented landscape of tools, evolving ethical requirements, emerging regulations, and rapidly shifting best practices. The first of two volumes, this book provides a comprehensive treatment of AI across the complete research lifecycle, from initial ideation through analysis, quality assurance, dissemination, and long-term impact.

Key Features:

- This book is the only resource covering AI applications across the entire research journey, from initial idea through long-term impact.
- It systematically applies four major AI governance frameworks (RUAIH, FUTURE-AI, NIST AI RMF, and GMLP) throughout both volumes, showing researchers how to operationalize abstract principles in daily practice.
- It includes detailed analysis of the EU AI Act implementation timeline (February 2025 through August 2027) with specific guidance for research applications. It helps researchers and institutions understand high-risk classifications, research exemptions, and compliance strategies before requirements take effect.
- It moves beyond hype and fear to deliver a balanced, practical approach to human–AI collaboration. Each chapter includes “Capabilities and Limitations”

analysis, ethical considerations, and implementation strategies that acknowledge both AI's transformative potential and its persistent limitations.

- This book features concrete examples demonstrating implementation principles in practice. Each chapter concludes with practical implementation strategies, reflection questions, and guidance applicable to institutions of varying sizes and resources.
- Volume 1 explores how AI can improve essential research activities, including designing studies, securing funding, navigating compliance and ethics reviews, recruiting participants, managing operations, collecting data, and analyzing results.
- Volume 2 continues the exploration of quality assurance, dissemination, peer review, impact, and the necessary institutional changes to responsibly implement AI capabilities.

AI for Biomedical Research Volume 1

From Idea to Analysis

Molly Klote

CRC Press
Taylor & Francis Group
Boca Raton London New York

CRC Press is an imprint of the
Taylor & Francis Group, an **informa** business

Designed cover image: Shutterstock

First edition published 2027
by CRC Press
2385 NW Executive Center Drive, Suite 320, Boca Raton FL 33431

and by CRC Press
4 Park Square, Milton Park, Abingdon, Oxon, OX14 4RN

CRC Press is an imprint of Taylor & Francis Group, LLC

ISBN: 9781041323426 (hbk)
ISBN: 9781041323396 (pbk)
ISBN: 9781003782995 (ebk)

DOI: 10.1201/9781003782995

Typeset in Times
by codeMantra

Contents

PART II Planning and Design

PART III Research Management and Administration

Book Information

Companion Volume: *AI for Biomedical Research Volume 2: Quality, Impact, and Implementation* (covering Research Integrity, Dissemination, Peer Review, Translation, Training, Infrastructure, ELSI, Implementation, and Future Directions)

Key Governance Frameworks Referenced

Throughout this volume, four key governance frameworks guide responsible AI use in research:

- RUAIH (Responsible Use of AI in Healthcare), Joint Commission/CHAI, 2025: Seven elements for healthcare AI governance
- FUTURE-AI, International consensus guideline, BMJ 2025: Six principles (Fairness, Universality, Traceability, Usability, Robustness, and Explainability)
- NIST AI RMF, National Institute of Standards and Technology, 2023: Four functions (Govern, Map, Measure, and Manage)
- GMLP (Good Machine Learning Practice), FDA/Health Canada/MHRA, 2021: Guiding principles for AI/ML in medical devices

These frameworks are introduced in Chapters 10, 13, and 14 and inform guidance throughout this book.

Preface

I have spent my career at the intersection of research and regulation, working to ensure that the pursuit of knowledge proceeds safely, ethically, and effectively. From my years at Walter Reed Army Medical Center to my work across 110 VA medical centers and to the HHS Office for Human Research Protections, I have witnessed firsthand both the transformative power of well-conducted research and the challenges that impede it. I have seen brilliant investigators struggle under administrative burdens, necessary studies delayed by inefficient processes, and critical questions go unasked because the path to answering them seemed too complex to navigate.

Throughout this work, I have been driven by a fundamental belief that the systems supporting research should enable rather than obstruct the scientific enterprise. When review processes are unclear or inconsistent, when administrative requirements consume researchers' time, when compliance becomes an end rather than a means, we all lose. Patients wait longer for treatment, communities go without the knowledge they need, and researchers grow frustrated with systems that seem designed to say "no" rather than "how can we get to yes?"

Technology has always promised to solve these challenges, but, until recently, that promise has largely gone unfulfilled. Early digitization efforts often automated existing inefficiencies, replacing paper forms with electronic ones without rethinking processes. We built systems that made researchers enter the same information multiple times, required manual interpretation of regulations that could be standardized, and relied on human memory to track complex compliance requirements across hundreds of active studies.

Artificial intelligence (AI) can represent something fundamentally different, not just automation but enhancement. AI can analyze large amounts of data to find patterns we might miss. It can maintain consistent standards across thousands of reviews while flagging cases that require human judgment. It can help match patients to research opportunities, researchers to funding sources, and institutions to best practices. Most importantly, when used thoughtfully, AI allows us to focus human expertise where it is most needed: on scientific and ethical questions that require wisdom, experience, and judgment.

My interest in AI is practical and hands-on. It stems from decades of working in research programs and compliance systems, spotting specific, real opportunities for improvement. I see AI as an opportunity across the entire research spectrum so I am documenting the applicability. The result is two complementary volumes. This volume, *AI for Biomedical Research Volume 1 From Idea to Analysis* throughout the book, outlines the full research process, from initial ideas through grant writing, literature review, study design, team assembly, compliance, ethics review, participant recruitment, operations, data collection, and analysis. The companion volume, *AI for Biomedical Research Volume 2: Quality, Impact, and Implementation*, focuses on what happens after analysis: ensuring research integrity, communicating and publishing findings, achieving translation and impact, training researchers, building infrastructure, navigating ethical and legal issues, implementing AI capabilities, and preparing for future challenges. Together, these two volumes offer a complete overview of AI throughout the entire research lifecycle.

This first volume explores how AI can improve essential research activities, including designing studies, securing funding, navigating compliance and ethics reviews, recruiting participants, managing operations, collecting data, and analyzing results. The companion volume continues the exploration of quality assurance, dissemination, peer review, impact, and the necessary institutional changes to responsibly implement AI capabilities. Both volumes target multiple audiences: researchers aiming to improve their work, administrators overseeing research operations, review board members assessing protocols, funders making strategic choices, and policymakers shaping the future of research.

Human and animal research protections remain central to my perspective throughout both volumes. AI tools must be developed and used in ways that address their rights and welfare, respect participant autonomy, protect privacy, promote equal participation, and maintain public trust in research. When discussing AI for participant recruitment, we need to consider informed consent and voluntary participation. When addressing AI for data analysis, we must focus on algorithmic bias and fairness. When evaluating AI for protocol review, we must ensure proper human oversight of ethical decisions. Technology reflects values; it does not replace them.

Throughout both volumes, I draw on emerging governance frameworks that provide essential guidance for responsible AI use: the Joint Commission and CHAI's Responsible Use of AI in Healthcare Framework, the international FUTURE-AI consensus guideline, the NIST AI Risk Management Framework, and the FDA's Good Machine Learning Practice principles. These frameworks, developed through extensive expert collaboration, offer practical guidance for navigating the opportunities and risks of AI in research contexts.

I also want to be realistic about what these volumes represent: a point-in-time primer in a rapidly evolving field. More capable systems will supersede the specific AI tools available as of this writing. Approaches that seem cutting-edge today will become standard practice. New applications will emerge that we cannot yet imagine. My goal is not to provide a comprehensive catalog of current AI tools; such a catalog would be obsolete before publication, but rather to establish frameworks for thinking about AI's role in research that will remain relevant even as specific technologies evolve.

If these volumes help researchers, administrators, and policymakers think more clearly about where and how AI can improve research, they will have served their purpose. If they contribute to AI being implemented thoughtfully rather than haphazardly, with appropriate attention to ethics and equity, they will have done important work. And if the field's experience with AI in research grows sufficiently that these books require updating with new insights, lessons learned, and emerging best practices, that will be the most tremendous success of all, because it will mean we are collectively learning how to leverage these powerful tools in the service of better science.

Research has always been a fundamentally human endeavor, driven by curiosity, creativity, and commitment to advancing knowledge for human benefit. AI will not change that fundamental nature. But it can help us conduct that human endeavor more effectively, more efficiently, and more equitably. That is the promise explored in this volume and its companion.

This book rejects the "black-box" approach to AI. Recognizing the documented risk of automation bias, I provide a structured "Human–AI–Human Sandwich" workflow for every stage of research. This ensures that the researcher remains the final arbiter of truth, equipped with specific "Override Protocols" to identify and correct AI hallucinations and biases.

THE "SANDWICH" IN PRACTICE: A SCIENTIFIC INTEGRITY AUDIT OF THESE VOLUMES

As a physician-researcher, I am acutely aware that recommending a "Human–AI–Human Sandwich" workflow is meaningless unless that workflow can withstand the rigors of scientific peer review. To that end, I have utilized these manuscripts as a living laboratory for the methods described in these chapters.

While large language models were utilized to assist in the structural organization, thematic synthesis, and initial drafting of this text, every word was subjected to the Override Protocols detailed in Chapter 1. This was not merely a matter of stylistic editing; it was a grueling process of clinical and regulatory fact-checking.

The necessity of the "Human-led Verification" phase, the top slice of the sandwich, is best illustrated by the data gathered during the writing of these books. My audit of the AI-generated outline of chapters revealed the following:

- **Reference Integrity**: Approximately 25% of all citations initially returned by the AI models were flawed.
- **The Hallucination Gap**: Roughly 3% of references were complete hallucinations with plausible-sounding titles and author lists for papers that do not exist in the physical or digital world.

- **The Accuracy Gap**: An additional 22% of citations contained significant errors, such as incorrect publication years, mismatched volume numbers, or the attribution of findings to the wrong authors.
- **Overlooked Content**: Approximately 12% of the topics ultimately included were overlooked by the initial AI outline.

Crucially, while the AI's conceptual summaries of the science were usually accurate, its ability to anchor those concepts in the historical record, the "receipts" of research, was demonstrably unreliable.

If I had accepted the AI's output without the final "Human" layer of the sandwich, these volumes would have contributed to the very "hallucination inflation" and "bias amplification" I warn against in Part III. Instead, the painstaking manual verification of 100% of the data points and citations herein serves as proof of this book's core argument:

AI does not replace the researcher's expertise; it demands a higher, more vigilant form of it. The "hostile editor" approach I applied to my own AI-assisted drafts is the same one I invite you to adopt as you integrate these tools into your research programs. The efficiency gained in the *Execution* phase (the middle of the sandwich) must always be reinvested into the *Verification* phase (the top of the sandwich). Scientific integrity in the age of AI is not found in the prompt; it is found in the audit.

I hope these volumes prove helpful in your work, whatever your role in the research enterprise. More than that, I hope they prompt reflection, discussion, and action to ensure that AI serves research and, through research, serves us all.

Dr. Molly Klote

Acknowledgments

I want to thank everyone who has helped me on my AI learning journey, including Craig Lipset, Angela Radcliffe, Jeffrey Ferraro, Rachel Ramoni, and Zak Kohane.

Thank you to my friends and family for supporting me as I took time away from events and gatherings to do this work.

Thank you to Perplexity (Claude Opus 4.6) and Gemini (Thinking) for helping me gather information and resources and for assisting me with drafting and editing this book so that it could be as up-to-date as possible when published.

About the Author

Molly Klote, MD, is the former Director of the US Department of Health and Human Services Office for Human Research Protections (OHRP). OHRP is the policy, education, and compliance office that oversees federally funded medical research for 21 federal agencies, 13,000 institutions, and over 6,000 institutional review boards in the United States and internationally. It is the proponent office for the policy known as "The Common Rule" (45 CFR 46). Before joining OHRP, Dr. Klote spent 6 years as the research policy, regulatory, and education lead for the Veterans Health Administration, the largest integrated healthcare system in the United States. Prior to the Veterans Health Administration, she served for 30 years in the Army, with her final assignment at the rank of Colonel, working for the Army Surgeon General, overseeing all US Army Human Research policy and compliance. Additionally, Dr. Klote has directed two major research program offices, served as an Institutional Official, chaired three Institutional Review Boards, and led a Research Scientific Review Board. She recently launched her own consulting company, Klote Medical Research Advisors, LLC, to bring her over 36 years of distinguished military and civilian federal experience to those who need to better understand federal research policy. She is the author of *Adapting to Change: Federal Policy Dynamics and the Pharmaceutical Industry*, 2025.

Part I

Foundations

1 Introduction to AI in Research

THE EVOLVING RESEARCH LANDSCAPE

Research has always been a human effort driven by curiosity, creativity, and the systematic pursuit of knowledge. For centuries, the fundamental process remained largely unchanged: researchers asked questions, designed studies, collected data, analyzed results, and shared their findings with communities. While tools evolved, from telescopes to electron microscopes, from paper notebooks to electronic databases, the core structure and workflow of research gradually changed.

The past 20 years have seen a swift increase in the speed and breadth of research, challenging traditional approaches. The volume of published literature roughly doubles every 17 years at a 4% compound annual growth rate, with over 3.4 million scientific papers released annually.[1] Research datasets have grown exponentially, from megabytes to petabytes and more.[2] Collaborations are happening more often across institutions, disciplines, and continents. Regulatory requirements have become more complex. Meanwhile, patient and community expectations for quick translation of research findings have strengthened.

This acceleration is fundamentally transforming the infrastructure of science. The AAAI 2025 Presidential Panel on the Future of AI Research, based on input from 25 leading researchers and a survey of 475 artificial intelligence (AI) community members, found that "the exponentially increasing quantity of AI research publications and the speed of AI innovation are testing the resilience of the peer-review system, with the immediate release of papers without peer-review evaluation having become

DOI 10.1201/9781003782995-2

widely accepted across many areas of AI research."[3] While the panel focused on AI as a discipline, its findings reflect a broader trend: across various fields, the growing volume of new knowledge is straining the systems researchers depend on to evaluate, synthesize, and build upon previous work.

These trends offer both opportunities and challenges. On the one side, we have unmatched access to data, computing power, and collaborative networks. On the other side, individual researchers and research teams struggle to keep up with the literature in their field, manage increasingly complex data, navigate bureaucratic regulations, and demonstrate the impact of their work in competitive funding environments.

Then AI arrives, a set of computational methods that can process large amounts of data, recognize patterns humans might miss, automate repetitive tasks, and improve human decision-making. AI is not science fiction or a distant future technology; it is here now, built into tools many researchers use every day without even noticing. When you use a citation manager that suggests relevant papers, rely on statistical software that finds anomalies in your data, or submit a manuscript to a journal that uses automated plagiarism detection, you are already working with AI.

What's changing is the scope, sophistication, and accessibility of AI applications throughout the entire research enterprise. AI is moving from isolated use cases to integration across the research lifecycle. It's shifting from tools that require specialized expertise to platforms accessible to any researcher. And it's evolving from systems that simply automate existing processes to ones that genuinely enhance human capabilities and enable new forms of research that weren't previously possible.

This transformation is neither automatic nor without challenges. AI tools are powerful but imperfect. They can reinforce biases in their training data. They may generate plausible-sounding but incorrect results. They require human oversight, critical thinking, and domain expertise to be used effectively. Recognizing where AI adds value and where it falls short is crucial for any researcher in today's environment.

WHAT RESEARCHERS NEED TO KNOW ABOUT AI

You don't need to be a computer scientist or a machine learning engineer to use AI effectively in your research. However, having a basic understanding of key concepts helps you evaluate AI tools, use them correctly, and avoid common mistakes.

HOW AI WORKS

At its core, AI refers to computer systems that can perform tasks usually requiring human intelligence: recognizing patterns, making predictions, understanding language, solving problems, and learning from experience. Modern AI includes several interconnected approaches.

Machine learning systems recognize patterns in data without explicitly being programmed with rules. Instead of telling a computer "if you see these specific characteristics, classify it as X," you give it thousands of examples and let it identify the key features.[4] This approach powers everything from spam filters to drug discovery platforms.

Natural language processing (NLP) allows computers to understand, interpret, and generate human language. NLP powers tools that summarize research articles, extract data from clinical notes, translate documents between languages, and assist with writing. Computer vision enables systems to analyze visual information from images and videos; in research settings, this includes examining microscopy images, identifying anomalies in medical scans, and extracting data from figures in published papers. Deep learning employs neural networks with multiple layers to learn hierarchical representations of data, achieving impressive success in tasks ranging from protein structure prediction[5] to generating human-like text, although these systems typically need substantial computational resources and training data.

Current large language models show how quickly these capabilities are improving. OpenAI's GPT-5 series, released in August 2025 with GPT-5.1 following in late 2025 (including variants like Instant, Thinking, Pro, and Codex-Max),[6] and Anthropic's Claude 4 family, which includes Claude Sonnet 4.6 released in

February 2026,[7] demonstrate advanced skills in reasoning, multimodal processing (text, images, and audio), and complex task execution. These models represent the cutting edge, but the field advances rapidly, and the specific systems available when you read this might differ from those described here, even as the core principles stay the same.

HOW AI LEARNS

Most modern AI systems learn by analyzing examples. A machine learning model designed to identify potential drug candidates doesn't rely on chemistry principles; instead, it learns from databases of known compounds and their properties. An NLP system that summarizes research papers learns from millions of texts and their human-written summaries.

This learning process has important implications for researchers. First, AI systems are only as good as their training data, if that data contains biases, gaps, or errors, the AI will likely reproduce them. This is not a metaphorical concern: a model trained mainly on clinical data from one demographic group will systematically perform worse on others. Second, AI systems work best on tasks similar to what they were trained on and may fail unpredictably in truly new situations. Third, more data generally leads to better outcomes, which is why AI has advanced most quickly in fields with abundant digital data.

Understanding these basics clarifies both AI's capabilities and its limitations. An AI trained on published research can quickly help you find relevant literature, but it cannot decide which research questions are truly worth pursuing. This depends on human judgment, values, and understanding of context. An AI can spot potential inconsistencies in your data, but it cannot determine whether they are errors, interesting anomalies, or new phenomena worth investigating.

KEY CONCEPTS

Several terms recur throughout this book and in the broader AI literature. An algorithm is a set of rules or procedures for solving a problem; in AI, algorithms define how systems process information and make decisions. Training data are the information used to teach an AI system, and its quality and representativeness fundamentally influence what the system learns. Validation is the process of testing an AI system on data it hasn't seen before to assess real-world performance, an essential step that distinguishes rigorous AI applications from unreliable ones. Bias refers to systematic errors or unfairness in AI outputs, often stemming from biases in training data or system design. A black box is an AI system whose internal decision-making is difficult or impossible to interpret, even for experts, posing challenges for trust and accountability in research settings where transparent, auditable methods are expected. Explainability is the extent to which an AI system's reasoning can be understood by humans. Generative AI refers to systems that produce new content, such as text, images, or code, rather than simply classifying or analyzing existing data. Lastly, hallucination describes when an AI system generates plausible-sounding but factually incorrect information, a common issue with large language models that makes verifying all AI outputs vital in research contexts.

FOUNDATIONAL AI CAPABILITIES AND LIMITATIONS FOR BIOMEDICAL RESEARCH

This section establishes the authoritative reference framework for the "Human–AI–Human Sandwich" methodology used throughout this book. While subsequent chapters provide domain-specific applications, the core capabilities and failure modes outlined here are the universal constraints of the current research ecosystem. To avoid redundancy, readers should refer to this Master Matrix as the baseline for expert supervision in all research phases.

This is not a convenience but a mandatory quality management system (Table 1.1).

THE HUMAN–AI–HUMAN SANDWICH: A GOVERNANCE FRAMEWORK

Efficiency in research is no longer defined by how fast one can write but by how rigorously one can audit. To maintain scientific

TABLE 1.1
The Master Capabilities and Limitations Matrix

Core Category	Research Application	AI Strength (The "Meat")	Potential Failure Mode	The Override Trigger
Semantic synthesis	Literature reviews; identifying research "white space"	Processing at scale; screening thousands of abstracts in seconds	**Contextual Drift:** Missing nuances in clinical guidelines or "hallucinating" consensus	When AI claims a "gold standard" exists, manual verification of guidelines is required
Narrative generation	Drafting grants, IRB protocols, and manuscripts	Rapidly producing structured first drafts and standardized reports	**Formulaic Bias:** Stripping away unique clinical "voice" and expert intuition	When drafting "Innovation" sections, human clinical "color" must be injected
Citation assembly	Locating and formatting references	Cross-referencing databases to build bibliographies	**The Hallucination Gap:** 3% fake citations; 22% incomplete/incorrect data	**Mandatory:** 1:1 manual check of every citation against a primary source (PubMed/DOI)
Pattern recognition	Anomaly detection in datasets; trend identification	Detecting subtle outliers in millions of observations	**Spurious Correlation:** Mistaking coincidental patterns for causal relationships	Any correlation suggested by AI must be vetted against known physiological or causal theory
Regulatory mapping	Cross-referencing FDA, OHRP, and NIST frameworks	Identifying overlaps between complex regulatory requirements	**Temporal Lag:** Missing the most recent 2026 executive orders or policy updates	When referencing "current" mandates; check actual.gov sites for the latest version
Code and scripting	Writing R/Python scripts for data analysis	Automating routine statistical calculations and data cleaning	**Logical Fragility:** Small library version errors leading to silent data corruption	Scripts handling raw clinical data must be peer-reviewed or tested with dummy data

The table serves as your primary guide for identifying when to delegate to AI and, more importantly, when to trigger a Manual Override.

integrity, we employ the Sandwich Workflow. This ensures AI is never the "start" or the "end" of the scientific process but a powerful engine wrapped in layers of clinical judgment.

1. **Initiation (Human)**: The researcher defines the clinical scope, ethical guardrails, and specific personas (e.g., "Act as a senior clinical trialist").
2. **Execution (AI)**: The AI performs the high-scale computational or drafting work, producing a *draft*, never a final product.
3. **Verification (The Override)**: The expert applies the Override Protocol, source validation, clinical sanity checks, and adversarial questioning, to transform "AI-generated" content into "Human-validated" evidence.

MOVING FROM THEORY TO APPLICATION

As I audited the creation of this very volume, I found that while AI was usually "conceptually right" in its drafts, its ability to ground those concepts in reality was unreliable (see the Preface for the 25% error-rate audit).

Each subsequent chapter in this book applies these general principles to specific research areas. To "kill the redundancy," from my initial draft of this volume, the Capabilities and Limitations sections in Chapters 2–15 will not reexplain *what* AI does; instead, they will focus exclusively on the Domain-Specific Override Triggers unique to that phase of research. Refer back to this Master Matrix whenever you encounter a new AI-assisted task to determine your specific verification responsibility.

MAPPING THE RESEARCH ECOSYSTEM

To understand where AI can be valuable, it helps to map the entire research lifecycle and its supporting infrastructure. Research is not a straight line but rather an interconnected ecosystem with multiple phases and stakeholders.

THE RESEARCH LIFECYCLE

The research lifecycle progresses through interconnected phases, each offering unique opportunities for AI support. The ideation phase marks the start, identifying key questions, unmet needs, and knowledge gaps through literature review, stakeholder consultation, trend analysis, and creative thinking about new approaches. The planning and design phase turns questions into studies, requiring suitable designs, resource planning, timeline estimation, budget creation, and team organization. The funding phase involves locating appropriate sources, preparing competitive proposals, navigating review processes, and managing awarded grants. The approval and compliance phase obtains necessary institutional permissions from institutional review boards (IRBs), Institutional Animal Care and Use Committee (IACUC), biosafety committees, and other oversight bodies, with ongoing compliance monitoring throughout the study.

For research involving human or animal subjects, the participant recruitment phase often involves the challenging task of identifying and enrolling suitable participants while ensuring diverse and representative samples. The operations phase manages activities, allocates resources, maintains quality, documents procedures, and ensures compliance, all while adapting to inevitable challenges and changes. The data management phase covers collection, cleaning, storage, security, and organization to ensure quality, privacy, and usability for analysis; increasingly, AI can also generate synthetic data that maintains statistical properties while protecting privacy, allowing data sharing, and enhancing limited datasets. The analysis phase involves applying appropriate methods to the data, with findings interpreted in light of existing knowledge and study limitations.

Throughout, integrity assurance systems maintain data integrity, detect potential misconduct, preserve audit trails, and uphold ethical standards. The dissemination phase shares findings via manuscripts, presentations, press releases, and channels tailored to different audiences. The publication phase involves peer review prior to formal publication, a process that is itself being reshaped by AI. In early 2026, Nature reported that AI tools are beginning to transform research assessment, sparking both enthusiasm and concern among academics about how AI-driven evaluation might reshape incentive structures, resource allocation, and the types of research valued.[8] The translation and impact phase ensures findings are implemented in practice, inform policy, enable new technologies, or advance fundamental knowledge. And training and capacity building occur throughout, as early-career researchers are developed and institutional research capacity is expanded.

SUPPORTING INFRASTRUCTURE

Research requires substantial infrastructure beyond the lifecycle itself: administrative systems for managing grants, contracts, compliance, and reporting; physical resources including laboratories, equipment, repositories, and computing infrastructure; human resources encompassing research teams, support staff, and collaborative networks; knowledge infrastructure such as libraries, databases, and knowledge management systems; and review and oversight systems like IRBs, IACUCs, safety committees, and data monitoring boards. AI has potential applications across all these phases and infrastructure components. Some are already well-developed; others present opportunities for future innovation.

HOW TO USE THIS BOOK

This book is designed to meet the needs of diverse audiences at different levels of engagement with AI.

For active researchers exploring any discipline, begin with chapters relevant to your current challenges, struggling with literature review? see Chapter 4; wrestling with participant recruitment? see Chapter 11. Pay special attention to the ethical considerations sections in each chapter, regardless of which AI tools you use. Explore chapters outside your immediate needs to uncover applications you might not have considered. For a thorough overview of ethical, legal, and social implications, implementation strategies, and future directions, refer to the companion volume, *AI for Biomedical Research Volume 2: Quality, Impact, and Implementation*.

For research administrators and leaders overseeing research programs, focusing on Chapters 6, 8–10, covering program optimization, administration, and regulatory review, along with the companion volume's chapters on infrastructure, implementation, and future directions, will aid in making strategic decisions about infrastructure and compliance.

For HRPP, IRB, and IACUC members, Chapters 9 and 10 specifically cover how AI can support your work and how to review AI-related protocols. The ethics principles section in this chapter offers essential context, and the companion volume explores ethical, legal, and social implications in greater detail.

For research staff and coordinators, chapters on compliance (8), recruitment (11), operations (12), and data management (13) will be most relevant to day-to-day challenges.

For funders and policymakers, review Chapter 6 on research portfolio optimization and Chapters 9 and 10 on oversight, with the companion volume providing in-depth coverage of translation, ethics, and future directions.

For students and trainees, this book explains how AI is transforming research careers. The companion volume features a dedicated training and education chapter, but all chapters here will help you understand the changing landscape you're entering.

A NOTE ON PACE OF CHANGE

AI is advancing quickly. The tools and capabilities discussed in this book may change, be replaced, or become outdated. However, the core principles, knowing where AI provides value, understanding its limits, and using it ethically and efficiently, will stay important even as specific technologies evolve. Instead of listing all current AI tools, this book emphasizes use cases, principles, and frameworks for assessing and applying AI within research. The aim is to offer lasting knowledge that helps you navigate AI's role in research, no matter which systems are available at any given time.

EMERGING GOVERNANCE FRAMEWORKS

As AI adoption in research accelerates, various governance frameworks have emerged to promote responsible development and deployment. These frameworks are complementary rather than competing, each focusing on different aspects of responsible AI usage.

International consensus frameworks offer the broadest guidance. The FUTURE-AI Consortium's 2025 guideline presents internationally recognized best practices based on six principles, Fairness, Universality, Traceability, Usability, Robustness, and Explainability, developed by 117 experts from 50 countries.[9] These principles are consistently referenced throughout this book as benchmarks for evaluating AI applications throughout the research lifecycle.

Risk management frameworks offer structured approaches to identifying and managing AI risks. The NIST AI Risk Management Framework (AI RMF 1.0) provides voluntary guidance through four core functions: Govern, Map, Measure, and Manage, creating a systematic approach applicable throughout the AI lifecycle.[10] The Map function helps organizations understand AI contexts and risks; the Measure function organizes performance assessment; and the Manage function guides mitigation and improvement.

Healthcare-specific guidance details the unique needs of clinical and health research environments. The Joint Commission and Coalition for Health AI created the Responsible Use of AI in Healthcare (RUAIH) framework, which includes seven key elements for healthcare organizations implementing AI tools, released in September 2025.[11]

Professional and regulatory guidance covers a wide range of approaches across different professional, regulatory, and geographic settings. The EU AI Act (Regulation 2024/1689), the first comprehensive AI legislation, categorizes AI systems used in healthcare and clinical research as "high risk," necessitating transparency requirements, conformity assessments, and increased oversight, with full enforcement for high-risk systems starting in August 2026.[12] The American Medical Association's policy on augmented intelligence and WHO regulatory considerations offer complementary strategies from professional and international health governance viewpoints.

Research community and publisher guidance address the practical realities of AI adoption in research settings. The AAAI 2025 Presidential Panel produced structured recommendations across 17 topics, including AI factuality, trustworthiness, and ethics, with over 75% of survey respondents rating factuality and trustworthiness as relevant or very relevant to their own research and 95% expressing interest in multidisciplinary approaches.[3] Emerging guidance from major publishers, including recommendations from Springer Nature's Korea Research Advisory Forum (KRAF) 2025, is helping institutions develop clear AI policies covering authorship, disclosure, peer review, and data governance.[13]

The speed of governance development mirrors the urgency of the challenge. In early 2026, Nature reported that AI is beginning to transform research assessment itself, raising both enthusiasm and concern about how AI-driven evaluation might reshape incentive structures, resource allocation, and the types of research that are valued.[8] These developments emphasize that governance is not a one-time task but an ongoing process that must adapt as AI capabilities and applications evolve.

FOUNDATIONAL ETHICAL PRINCIPLES FOR AI IN RESEARCH

The governance frameworks described above provide structural guidance for responsible AI deployment. However, frameworks operate within a deeper ethical foundation, the principles that explain why certain uses of AI are acceptable and others are not. This section outlines the ethical principles that recur throughout this book.

HISTORICAL FOUNDATIONS

Research ethics did not develop in isolation. The Belmont Report (1978) introduced three core principles, respect for persons, beneficence, and justice, that have directed human subjects research for nearly 50 years.[14] These principles were responses to specific harms: research conducted without informed consent, studies that put participants at unacceptable risks, and investigations that systematically targeted vulnerable populations while advantaging the privileged.

AI in research presents similar concerns in new ways. When an AI system handles participant data, what must informed consent include? When an algorithm makes decisions impacting research participants, how is beneficence evaluated? When AI tools behave differently across demographic groups, what does justice require? The Belmont principles remain completely relevant, but applying them requires adaptation for an AI context.

NIST's Belmont-AI initiative has started this translation, highlighting additional considerations such as explainability, privacy, reliability, and security that expand the Belmont framework for AI applications.[15] The challenge isn't replacing established ethical principles but enhancing them to address capabilities and risks that the original creators could not have foreseen.

CORE ETHICAL PRINCIPLES FOR AI IN RESEARCH

Seven principles form the ethical foundation for using AI in research settings. These build on and expand the frameworks mentioned earlier, combining core research ethics with AI-specific considerations.

Transparency and disclosure require that the use of AI in research be openly acknowledged and documented. Researchers should reveal when and how they use AI tools in their work, including in publications, grant applications, and regulatory submissions. AI systems employed in research should be well-documented so that their capabilities, limitations, and potential biases can be assessed. Additionally, the rationale behind AI-assisted decisions should be understandable, not necessarily that every algorithmic step can be traced, but that the reasoning for using AI, its contribution, and the basis for trusting its outputs can be explained and justified.

Accountability and oversight require that humans stay responsible for research decisions, even when AI tools influence those choices. Clear accountability should be assigned for AI-assisted decisions, with specific individuals overseeing the process. Sufficient human review of AI outputs must be maintained, adjusted according to the stakes involved, and more rigorous reviews for high-stakes applications. Additionally, systems for detecting, reporting, and fixing AI errors should be put in place before deployment, not after issues arise.

Fairness and equity require that AI systems used in research do not systematically disadvantage any group. AI tools should be evaluated for differential performance across demographic groups, with special attention to populations historically underrepresented in research. AI should not perpetuate or amplify existing biases in research processes, from participant selection to peer review. Additionally, AI tools should be accessible to researchers with varying levels of resources, preventing AI from widening rather than narrowing existing inequalities in the research field. As Barucci and colleagues note in their 2026 European perspective on the AI Act's implications for clinical research, particular attention must be paid to ensuring that AI-driven systems do not worsen disparities in who benefits from and who bears the risks of clinical research.[16]

Privacy and data protection require that AI systems used in research respect participant privacy and comply with data protection laws. Data used for training or operating AI should be collected and used with informed consent and in accordance with applicable regulations. AI features that could enable reidentification of anonymized data or inference of sensitive attributes need specific safeguards. Additionally, data governance frameworks should address the unique risks posed by AI, such as model memorization of training data and the potential for AI to extract information beyond what participants agreed to share.

Beneficence and nonmaleficence require that AI use in research aims to benefit participants, communities, and science while minimizing potential harms. The benefits of AI should be balanced against risks, including errors, bias, and unintended consequences. AI should enhance rather than replace the human elements of research that protect participants, judgment, empathy, and ethical reasoning that safeguard welfare. Additionally, potential harms from AI, including those to participants, researchers, communities, and the integrity of science, should be actively identified and mitigated.

Scientific integrity requires that AI use strengthens rather than weakens the rigor and trustworthiness of research. AI tools should improve reproducibility through systematic documentation and consistent application of methods. AI-generated content (text, data, and analyses) should be clearly identified and verified. The limitations of AI analyses, including potential biases, failure modes, and uncertainty, should be honestly disclosed. Additionally, AI should not be used to fabricate, falsify, or misrepresent research data or findings, especially as generative AI makes fabrication easier and detection more difficult. Findings from Springer Nature's KRAF 2025 show that researchers who have experimented with AI tools nearly all find them helpful, yet many institutions have not established the AI policies, disclosure standards, or training programs needed to ensure that this helpfulness promotes integrity rather than shortcuts.[13]

Respect for human agency means that AI should support, not replace, human decision-making in research. Researchers must keep meaningful control over the research process, even when AI manages operational tasks. Participants should be aware when AI is involved in research that impacts them. Additionally, the development and use of AI tools should honor the expertise, judgment, and values of the researchers and communities involved.

APPLYING THESE PRINCIPLES

These seven principles are not mere abstract goals; they serve as practical guides for the everyday decisions researchers encounter. When a researcher considers using an AI tool to screen potential study participants, transparency requires disclosing the AI's role in the consent process; fairness involves assessing whether the tool performs equally across demographic groups; accountability requires a human to review the AI's choices before finalizing enrollment decisions. When a research team employs generative AI to draft a section of a manuscript, scientific integrity demands verifying each factual claim; transparency involves disclosing the AI's contribution; and respect for human agency requires that the researchers, not the AI, determine the scientific arguments and conclusions.

Each subsequent chapter contains an ethical considerations section that applies these core principles to specific research contexts. Those sections assume familiarity with the principles outlined here and focus on domain-specific ethical challenges rather than reexplaining the general framework.

LOOKING AHEAD

The following chapters examine AI applications throughout every stage of the research lifecycle. Each chapter follows a similar format: defining the challenge, explaining how AI addresses it, discussing current capabilities, acknowledging limitations, and exploring ethical considerations.

Research has always centered on enhancing human abilities; we use microscopes to see what our eyes cannot, telescopes to observe distant phenomena, and statistical methods to understand complex patterns. AI is the next step in this tradition of creating tools that expand human capability. When used carefully, it can help us ask better questions, conduct more rigorous studies, and interpret findings more thoughtfully.

The keyword is "thoughtfully." AI is neither a savior nor a threat but a powerful tool that requires human judgment, domain expertise, and ethical reasoning to be used effectively. This book aims to equip you with the knowledge to use AI thoughtfully to advance your research.

KEY TAKEAWAYS

- AI is transforming every stage of the research cycle, from ideation to impact assessment, not as a future option but as a current reality embedded in tools many researchers already use.

- AI excels at large-scale processing, pattern recognition, enforcing consistency, automating routine tasks, and synthesizing knowledge, tasks involving volume, speed, and systematic application of criteria.
- AI performs poorly in judgment, ethical reasoning, contextual interpretation, causal understanding, creative insight, relationship building, and deliberative discussion, the essential human elements of research.
- The human–AI partnership model is the most effective approach: AI manages computational complexity while humans contribute scientific reasoning, ethical judgment, and contextual interpretation.
- All AI outputs need verification, hallucinations, brittleness, training data dependence, and black-box opacity make uncritically accepting AI outputs unacceptable in research contexts.
- Multiple governance frameworks (FUTURE-AI, NIST AI RMF, RUAIH, and EU AI Act) offer complementary guidance for responsible AI deployment in research.
- Seven ethical principles, transparency, accountability, fairness, privacy, beneficence, scientific integrity, and respect for human agency, form the foundation for responsible AI use throughout the research lifecycle.
- The speed of AI development means certain tools will evolve, but the core principles for evaluating and implementing AI responsibly will remain the same.

QUESTIONS FOR REFLECTION

1. Where in your research workflow can AI offer the greatest value, and which aspects of human judgment will still be essential even with AI help?
2. How would you verify AI outputs in your specific research context, what domain knowledge and validation methods would you use?
3. Which of the seven ethical principles do you find most difficult to apply in your research setting, and why?

4. How ready is your institution to support responsible AI adoption, what policies, training, and governance structures are in place or needed?
5. How might AI tools influence equity in your field, could they reduce or increase existing gaps between well-resourced and resource-limited researchers?

NOTES

1. Bornmann, L., & Mutz, R. (2015). Growth rates of modern science: A bibliometric analysis based on the number of publications and cited references. *Journal of the Association for Information Science and Technology*, 66(11), 2215–2222. https://doi.org/10.1002/asi.23329. Note: Foundational bibliometric analysis establishing the ~4% compound annual growth rate of scientific publications and the approximately 17-year doubling time that characterizes the exponential expansion of the research literature.
2. Hey, T., et al. (2009). *The Fourth Paradigm: Data-Intensive Scientific Discovery*. Microsoft Research. https://www.microsoft.com/en-us/research/publication/fourth-paradigm-data-intensive-scientific-discovery/. Note: Influential framing of data-intensive science as the "fourth paradigm" of research (after empirical, theoretical, and computational approaches), presciently documenting the exponential growth of research data that would accelerate further in the following decade.
3. Rossi, F., et al. (2025). AAAI 2025 presidential panel on the future of AI research: report. Association for the Advancement of Artificial Intelligence. https://aaai.org/about-aaai/presidential-panel-on-the-future-of-ai-research/. Note: Comprehensive report drawing on input from 25 leading researchers and 475 survey respondents, covering 17 topics including factuality (identified as the single largest topic in AI research), trustworthiness, ethics, and the role of academia.
4. Vamathevan, J., et al. (2019). Applications of machine learning in drug discovery and development. *Nature Reviews Drug Discovery*, 18(6), 463–477. https://doi.org/10.1038/s41573-019-0024-5. Note: Comprehensive review of ML applications across the drug discovery pipeline, illustrating how pattern-learning approaches have transformed pharmaceutical research from target identification through clinical development.

5. Jumper, J., et al. (2021). Highly accurate protein structure prediction with AlphaFold. *Nature*, 596(7873), 583–589. https://doi.org/10.1038/s41586-021-03819-2. Note: AlphaFold's demonstration that deep learning could predict protein 3D structures with near-experimental accuracy represents one of the most consequential AI achievements in scientific research, earning the 2024 Nobel Prize in Chemistry.
6. OpenAI. (2025). GPT-5/GPT-5.1 model family. https://openai.com/index/introducing-gpt-5/; https://openai.com/index/introducing-gpt-5-1/. Note: The GPT-5 series (August 2025) and GPT-5.1 (late 2025, variants: Instant, Thinking, Pro, Codex-Max) represent the current frontier of large language model capabilities, with significant advances in reasoning, multimodal processing, and complex task execution.
7. Anthropic. (2026). Claude Sonnet 4.6. https://www.anthropic.com/news/claude-sonnet-4-6. Note: Released February 2026, Claude Sonnet 4.6 demonstrates continued rapid advancement in LLM capabilities including enhanced reasoning and multimodal processing.
8. Nature. (2026, February 4). AI could transform research assessment, and some academics are worried. DOI: 10.1038/d41586-026-00124-8. Note: Reports on the emerging use of AI in research evaluation, documenting both enthusiasm for efficiency gains and concern about how AI-driven assessment might reshape incentive structures and which research is valued.
9. Lekadir, K., et al. (2025). FUTURE-AI: International consensus guideline for trustworthy and deployable artificial intelligence in healthcare. *The BMJ*, 388, e081554. https://doi.org/10.1136/bmj-2024-081554. Note: International consensus developed by 117 experts from 50 countries, establishing six core principles (Fairness, Universality, Traceability, Usability, Robustness, and Explainability) for trustworthy AI. Referenced throughout this book as a touchstone framework.
10. National Institute of Standards and Technology. (2023). Artificial Intelligence Risk Management Framework (AI RMF 1.0). NIST AI 100-1. https://www.nist.gov/itl/ai-risk-management-framework. Note: Voluntary risk management framework organized around four functions (Govern, Map, Measure, and Manage) providing structured approaches to AI risk identification and mitigation throughout the lifecycle.

11. The Joint Commission & Coalition for Health AI. (2025). Responsible Use of AI in Healthcare (RUAIH). https://digitalassets.jointcommission.org/api/public/content/dcfcf4f1a0cc45cdb526b3cb034c68c2. Note: Released September 17, 2025, RUAIH provides seven key elements for healthcare organizations implementing AI, addressing governance, clinical validation, transparency, and ongoing monitoring.
12. European Parliament and Council of the European Union. (2024). Regulation (EU) 2024/1689 laying down harmonised rules on artificial intelligence (AI Act). *Official Journal of the European Union*. https://artificialintelligenceact.eu. Note: The first comprehensive AI legislation globally, classifying AI systems by risk level with specific requirements for high-risk applications including those in healthcare and clinical research. Full applicability for high-risk systems begins August 2026.
13. Kim, H. (2026). Fostering Responsible AI Use in Research and Publishing: Insights from the Korea Research Advisory Forum (KRAF) 2025. *Springer Nature*. Note: Documents findings from KRAF 2025 that researchers who experiment with AI tools almost universally find them helpful, while institutions lag in developing the AI policies, disclosure standards, and training programs needed for responsible adoption, a gap with significant implications for research integrity.
14. National Commission for the Protection of Human Subjects of Biomedical and Behavioral Research. (1979). The Belmont Report: Ethical Principles and Guidelines for the Protection of Human Subjects of Research. U.S. Department of Health and Human Services. https://www.hhs.gov/ohrp/regulations-and-policy/belmont-report/. Note: Foundational document establishing respect for persons, beneficence, and justice as the three core principles for ethical research involving human subjects.
15. Greene, T., et al. (2024). Extending the Belmont Report to AI Research. NIST. Note: NIST initiative translating the Belmont Report's principles for AI contexts, identifying additional considerations including explainability, privacy, reliability, and security that extend the original framework.
16. Barucci, A., et al. (2026). Ethical and regulatory frameworks for artificial intelligence in clinical research: A European perspective. *European Cardiology Review*, 21, e01. https://pmc.ncbi.nlm.nih.gov/articles/PMC12888102/. Note: Published January 2026, provides a European perspective on the AI Act's implications for clinical research ethics, with particular attention to equity, informed consent in AI contexts, and ensuring AI-driven systems do not exacerbate research disparities.

Part II

Planning and Design

2 AI for Biomedical Research Ideation and Planning

THE CHALLENGE OF RESEARCH IDEATION

Every research project begins with a question, but not all questions are created equal. Some lead to transformative discoveries that reshape entire fields. Others, despite consuming substantial resources, yield incremental findings with limited impact. Still others, however well-intentioned, prove infeasible due to technical limitations, insufficient resources, or lack of necessary expertise.

Identifying research opportunities that are important, new, and achievable is one of the most difficult parts of a researcher's work. It requires:

Comprehensive awareness of what has already been discovered and what questions remain unanswered. With over 3.4 million scientific papers published annually across all disciplines,[1] maintaining current awareness has become nearly impossible through traditional methods. As the AAAI 2025 Presidential Panel documented, the sheer volume and pace of new research is straining peer-review systems and making it increasingly common for findings to circulate without formal evaluation.[2]

Recognition of emerging trends before they become obvious to everyone. The researchers who identify important questions early often secure competitive advantages in funding and publication.[3] But spotting nascent trends requires synthesizing information across disparate sources and disciplines.

Understanding the needs of stakeholders that research can address. For translational and applied research, it is crucial to

DOI 10.1201/9781003782995-4

understand the specific problems faced by patients, clinicians, policymakers, or communities. However, researchers often work in relative isolation from end users.

Realistic evaluation of feasibility considering available resources, current technology, regulatory limits, and timeline needs. Many promising research ideas fail not because the science is wrong but because researchers underestimate practical barriers.

Identifying the complementary expertise needed to address complex questions. Modern research increasingly demands interdisciplinary teams, but finding the right collaborators across traditional boundaries remains a challenge.

Understanding funding landscapes and aligning research interests with funder priorities are crucial. Even excellent research ideas need financial support, and knowing what funding opportunities are available takes time.

Traditionally, research ideation relies heavily on individual researchers' knowledge, intuition, and networks. Senior researchers draw on years of experience and extensive professional connections. Early-career researchers often face these challenges, possibly missing important opportunities or chasing questions that more experienced colleagues would see as problematic.

Artificial intelligence (AI) is starting to transform this landscape by enabling systematic analysis of large volumes of information, uncovering patterns across disciplines, and revealing connections that might otherwise stay hidden. This chapter explores how.

IDENTIFYING RESEARCH OPPORTUNITIES AND GAPS

The first step in research ideation is recognizing what we don't know, identifying gaps in current knowledge that present opportunities for investigation.

SYSTEMATIC LITERATURE ANALYSIS

AI-powered tools can now analyze entire bodies of literature to identify understudied areas, contradictory findings, and emerging questions. Unlike traditional literature reviews conducted by individual researchers examining dozens or hundreds of papers, AI systems can process tens of thousands of publications to map knowledge landscapes. Tools such as Elicit, Semantic Scholar, and Scispace now give researchers the ability to perform systematic gap analysis across large bodies of literature, extracting key concepts, identifying understudied intersections, and surfacing contradictory findings, capabilities that were impractical just a few years ago.[4]

GAP IDENTIFICATION APPROACHES

Natural language processing algorithms can extract key concepts, methods, and findings from published papers and then identify combinations of concepts that occur frequently versus those that are rare or missing. For example, if research extensively covers "condition X in population A" and "condition X in population B" but rarely mentions "condition X in population C," this indicates a possible gap.

Citation network analysis can identify areas where multiple research streams converge without clear integration, highlighting opportunities for combined efforts. Conversely, it can detect topics that garner few citations despite seeming significance, potentially pointing to high-impact gaps.

Temporal analysis reveals which questions have been answered recently and which ones remain open for a long time. Long-standing unanswered questions may either be very challenging problems needing new methods or overlooked opportunities.

PRACTICAL APPLICATIONS

A cancer researcher might use AI to analyze oncology literature and discover that, while immunotherapy has been extensively studied in melanoma and lung cancer, some rare tumor types remain largely unexplored, presenting opportunities for translational research.

An education researcher might recognize that, although online learning has been extensively studied in university settings, questions about how it is implemented in rural K-12 schools still remain understudied despite their policy importance.

A materials scientist might find that while certain classes of compounds are well characterized, the combinations of properties useful for specific applications haven't been systematically studied.

CROSS-DISCIPLINARY CONNECTION DISCOVERY

Some of the most innovative research comes from linking ideas across normally separate fields. AI is great at spotting these possible connections by analyzing literature from different areas.

Mechanism Discovery: AI can recognize similar mechanisms or approaches used in different fields that might be adaptable. For example, machine learning techniques developed for image recognition in computer science have applications in medical imaging, materials characterization, and ecological monitoring.

Analogous Problems: AI can recognize when seemingly different fields face structurally similar challenges. Game theory, originally developed in economics, has found applications in evolutionary biology, computer science, and international relations. AI can help identify new domains where existing analytical frameworks might apply.[5]

Complementary Methods: Researchers in one field may be unaware of methodological advances in adjacent disciplines. AI can surface relevant techniques by analyzing methodological descriptions across papers, even when the domains seem unrelated.

CONTRADICTORY FINDINGS AND REPLICATION OPPORTUNITIES

Scientific progress depends on reconciling conflicting results. AI can systematically identify papers reporting contradictory findings on similar questions, highlighting either replication opportunities or conditions where results differ.

For example, AI analysis might reveal that studies of a particular intervention show positive effects in some populations but not others, with the difference potentially relating to demographic factors, implementation fidelity, or measurement approaches. This creates opportunities for research explicitly designed to understand moderating factors.

Similarly, AI can identify highly cited findings that have never been independently replicated, a concern that has gained renewed importance. The original 2015 Reproducibility Project in psychology found that only about 36% of studied findings could be successfully replicated.[6] In 2025, the reproducibility debate intensified when a presidential executive order specifically highlighted a "reproducibility crisis" in science, and proposals emerged for the National Institutes of Health (NIH) to allocate at least $48 million annually to fund replication studies.[7] While scientists debate whether the term "crisis" accurately describes the situation, Brian Nosek, who led the original replication effort, notes that "if we define a crisis as something that's changing for the worse, we don't have the evidence to say that's happening," there is broad agreement that systematic replication of key findings presents an important research opportunity. AI can help identify which high-impact findings most urgently need replication by analyzing citation networks, methodological vulnerabilities, and the extent to which downstream research relies on unreplicated results.

TREND ANALYSIS AND EMERGING TOPICS

Beyond identifying current gaps, AI can help researchers anticipate where their fields are heading and position themselves to contribute to emerging areas.

PUBLICATION TREND ANALYSIS

By analyzing publication rates, citation patterns, and funding allocations over time, AI can identify topics gaining momentum versus those plateauing or declining.

Early trend detection: Instead of waiting for a topic to become mainstream, AI can spot rising interest patterns. For example, analysis might reveal that publications on a specific subject are growing at 30% annually over 3 years, with citation rates increasing as well, indicating an emerging area where early involvement could be beneficial.

Lifecycle Analysis: Different research topics follow predictable lifecycles: emergence, rapid growth, maturity, and sometimes decline. Understanding where a potential research area fits in this lifecycle helps inform strategic decisions. Entering a mature field requires a different approach than entering an emerging one.

Geographic and Institutional Patterns: AI can identify where specific research topics are most prominent, which countries, institutions, or research groups are leading in particular fields. This information helps researchers find potential collaborators, understand competitive landscapes, and see where their unique perspectives could add value.

SOCIAL MEDIA AND PREPRINT ANALYSIS

Published literature reflects the final stage of research, often appearing months or years after the initial work. AI analysis of preprints, conference proceedings, and social media activity related to research offers earlier signals of emerging trends.

Preprint servers like arXiv, bioRxiv, and medRxiv have become a significant force in scientific communication. Approximately 14% of published biomedical research first appears as preprints, with bioRxiv and medRxiv together attracting 10 million visitors each month.[8] By the end of 2025, bioRxiv and medRxiv will host over 389,000 preprints, with bioRxiv alone posting 49,256 new manuscripts in 2025, its busiest year on record.[9] AI can analyze preprint trends to identify topics gaining attention 6–12 months before they appear in peer-reviewed journals.

Analysis of scientific conferences, examining abstracts, keynote topics, and participant discussions, offers additional early indicators. What is featured prominently at major conferences often forecasts publication trends in the following years.

Research-focused social media activity, such as Twitter/X discussions among scientists, blog posts, and online forums, can reveal emerging controversies, questions, and approaches even earlier in their development.

GRANT AND FUNDING TREND ANALYSIS

Funding agency priorities both influence and guide research directions. AI analysis of awarded grants offers insights into the questions funders deem important and the approaches they are willing to support.

By examining grant titles, abstracts, and funding amounts over time, AI can identify:

- New program announcements and funding mechanisms
- Shifts in priority areas within agencies
- Successful framing and positioning of proposals in emerging areas
- Decline in funding for specific topics or approaches

This information helps researchers match their interests with funding opportunities and predict future chances.

TECHNOLOGY AND METHODS EMERGENCE

New research opportunities often emerge from technological advances or methodological innovations. AI can monitor the progress and adoption of new technologies and methods across different fields.

For example, the development of CRISPR gene editing,[10] single-cell sequencing,[11] or large language models (LLMs)[12] has created new research opportunities. AI analysis of methods sections in papers can identify when new techniques are shifting from specialized labs to broader use, a sign that the necessary infrastructure and expertise are becoming accessible for researchers.

STAKEHOLDER AND COMMUNITY NEEDS ASSESSMENT

Research has impact when it tackles questions that matter to stakeholders outside academia. AI can assist researchers in understanding and prioritizing problems that patients, clinicians, policymakers, or communities actually encounter.

PATIENT AND COMMUNITY VOICE ANALYSIS

Understanding health priorities from patient perspectives has traditionally depended on focus groups, surveys, and advisory boards, important methods but often slow and with limited reach.

AI can enhance these methods by analyzing patient forums, support group discussions, social media conversations, and patient-reported outcome databases to identify common concerns, unmet needs, and questions.[13]

Important Ethical Considerations: This type of analysis must be conducted carefully to protect privacy, prevent exploitation, and ensure findings inform rather than replace direct community engagement. Analyzing public forums differs from analyzing private medical data, as the former is generally more suitable for identifying broad themes while respecting individual privacy.

EXAMPLE APPLICATIONS

A researcher studying diabetes management might analyze patient forum discussions to find that while clinical trials mainly focus on glucose control, patients consistently show more concern about hypoglycemia fear, the cost of supplies, and how it affects their jobs. This could help set research priorities.

Mental health researchers might discover, through analysis of support group discussions, that people with specific conditions consistently report that existing treatments don't target certain symptoms, highlighting opportunities for developing new therapies.

CLINICAL PRACTICE GAP IDENTIFICATION

For clinical and translational research, understanding the gaps between evidence and practice is essential. AI can analyze electronic health records (with proper privacy protections), clinical guidelines, and actual prescribing or treatment patterns to identify discrepancies.

Where clinical guidelines recommend specific approaches but actual practice varies significantly, this indicates either implementation barriers worth exploring or situations where guidelines may not align with clinical realities.

Similarly, analysis can identify circumstances where treatment variability is very high, indicating either a lack of evidence or complexity that evidence-based guidelines do not sufficiently address. Both situations present research opportunities.

POLICY AND SOCIETAL CHALLENGE ANALYSIS

For research aimed at informing policy, understanding the questions policymakers truly face is crucial. AI can examine policy documents, legislative testimony, regulatory filings, and public comments to find common questions and areas where knowledge is lacking.

For example, analyzing environmental policy documents might highlight common questions about the cost-effectiveness of specific interventions, challenges in implementation within certain contexts, or gaps in monitoring capabilities, all of which present clear research opportunities with policy relevance.

INDUSTRY AND TECHNOLOGY NEEDS

For research with commercial uses, understanding industry challenges and technology gaps helps identify opportunities. AI can analyze patent filings, industry reports, corporate research publications, and market analyses to find problems companies are trying to solve.

Areas with many patents filed but few cited or commercialized may signal particularly challenging problems where academic research can provide fundamental insights.

FEASIBILITY ANALYSIS AND RESOURCE ESTIMATION

Identifying an important question is only the first step. Research must also be feasible based on available resources, technology, expertise, and time.

RESOURCE REQUIREMENT PREDICTION

AI can analyze similar completed projects to estimate resource needs for proposed research. By reviewing grants, publications, and project reports from comparable studies, AI can provide data-driven estimates of:

Timeline Requirements: How long did similar projects take from start to finish? What factors (sample size, methodology complexity, regulatory requirements) are associated with longer or shorter timelines?

Budget Needs: What were the costs of comparable studies? How have expenses evolved over time? What are typical budget allocations for personnel, equipment, supplies, and other categories?

Personnel Requirements: What size teams conducted similar work? What expertise was represented? How many staff hours were allocated?

Infrastructure Needs: What facilities, equipment, or technical capabilities were required for similar projects?

These estimates help researchers determine whether proposed projects align with available resources or require additional support.

TECHNICAL FEASIBILITY ASSESSMENT

Some research questions, although important, might not be technically feasible with current methods or technology. AI can assist in evaluating feasibility by:

Method Availability Analysis: Assessing whether necessary measurement techniques, analytical methods, or experimental approaches are available and accessible.

Technology Maturity Assessment: Determining whether the necessary technologies are established and dependable or still under development.

Successful Precedent Identification: Determining whether anyone has successfully carried out similar approaches and, if so, in what contexts.

Barrier Identification: Identifying technical challenges faced by earlier research efforts.

For example, a researcher proposing to measure specific biomarkers might use AI to identify whether validated assays are available, what sample requirements are, and whether earlier studies have successfully employed these measurements in their target population.

REGULATORY AND ETHICAL FEASIBILITY

Research involving human subjects, animals, controlled substances, or export-controlled technologies is subject to regulatory requirements that affect feasibility. AI can assist researchers in understanding likely regulatory pathways by analyzing:

Similar Approved Protocols: What requirements did comparable studies fulfill? What review processes did they go through?

Regulatory Precedents: How have review boards or agencies managed similar research questions or methods?

Ethical Considerations: What ethical concerns have been raised about similar work, and how were they addressed?

This analysis helps researchers anticipate regulatory requirements early in the planning process, preventing proposals that could encounter insurmountable barriers. For research involving AI systems themselves, the EU AI Act's classification of healthcare AI as "high risk" (discussed in Chapter 1) may introduce additional compliance planning needs to be considered during feasibility assessment.

RISK ASSESSMENT

All research involves some level of risk, such as hypotheses being unsupported, methods failing, or results ending up inconclusive. AI can assist in assessing these risks by analyzing:

Success Rates: For similar research questions or methods, what percentage of studies yielded definitive results compared to inconclusive findings?
Common Failure Points: Where have similar projects faced issues? Were there recurring patterns in what went wrong?
Contingency Needs: Did successful projects require backup plans or alternative strategies?

This doesn't mean avoiding risky research, transformative work often requires taking chances. But it means taking risks with awareness and proper mitigation strategies.

AI-ASSISTED HYPOTHESIS GENERATION

Beyond pinpointing gaps and trends, AI is increasingly being used to generate research hypotheses directly. Early evidence suggests this capability is real but requires careful human evaluation.

A 2025 study in the *Journal of Medical Internet Research* examined GPT-4o's ability to generate research hypotheses for cardiotoxicity research.[14] The AI generated 96 hypotheses across five challenge areas, with 14% rated as highly novel and 65% as moderately novel by expert evaluators. Importantly, literature searches revealed existing publications for only 29% of the hypotheses, indicating genuine novelty in most cases. However, when the AI created detailed experimental plans for the most promising hypotheses, evaluators found the plans were "often deemed overly ambitious, highlighting the need for more practical considerations."[14]

This pattern, strong performance in generating creative hypotheses but weaker performance in practical planning, highlights the human–AI partnership model described in Chapter 1.

AI can broaden the range of possibilities researchers consider, but human domain expertise remains crucial for assessing feasibility, prioritizing options, and turning promising ideas into actionable research plans. Google's AI coscientist, introduced in early 2025, adopts a more structured approach by using specialized agents that iteratively generate, debate, and refine hypotheses, but even this system is meant to support rather than replace human scientific judgment.[15]

GRANT OPPORTUNITY MATCHING

Even well-conceived, feasible research requires funding. The grant landscape is vast and constantly evolving, making it difficult for researchers to identify all relevant opportunities.

FUNDING SOURCE DISCOVERY

AI can continuously monitor funding announcements from government agencies, private foundations, industry sources, and international organizations, matching opportunities to researcher profiles and interests. Tools like Be$tMatch, developed at West Virginia University, use LLMs to analyze NIH Notices of Funding Opportunity and match them to faculty research profiles, delivering personalized notifications every 2 weeks.[16] Similar platforms are emerging from commercial providers, offering automated opportunity scanning across multiple funding databases.

Active Matching: Using a researcher's publication history, interests, and institutional profile, AI can identify and notify researchers of relevant funding opportunities as they are announced.

Passive Discovery: Instead of waiting for announcements, AI can analyze funding trends to forecast when new opportunities may arise. If an agency funds similar programs every 3–4 years, AI can identify when a new round might be expected.

Hidden Opportunities: Some funding sources are not widely advertised but are listed in agency budgets, strategic plans, or administrative documents. AI can help identify these less obvious opportunities.

FUNDER PRIORITY ALIGNMENT

Understanding what funders truly prioritize, beyond their stated objectives, helps researchers position their proposals effectively. AI can analyze:

Funded Project Characteristics: What types of projects actually received funding compared to what the opportunity announcement emphasized? Sometimes funder priorities differ from the language of the announcement.

Success Factors: Among similar proposals, which characteristics were linked to funding? Specific methods, collaborative structures, or framing approaches?

Reviewer Expertise: Who reviewed similar proposals, and what are their backgrounds and interests? This helps researchers tailor proposals to potential reviewer audiences.

Budget Patterns: What budget ranges do specific funding mechanisms usually support? What aspects do funded budgets emphasize?

COLLABORATIVE FUNDING OPPORTUNITIES

Many funding opportunities either require or prefer collaboration across institutions, disciplines, or sectors. AI can assist in identifying:

- Which institutions frequently partner on funded projects
- What types of collaborations particular funders value
- Potential partners with complementary expertise and track records
- Required versus optional collaboration structures

This information helps researchers form teams aligned with funder preferences.

INTERDISCIPLINARY RESEARCH DISCOVERY

Many crucial research questions require combining knowledge and methods from different disciplines. However, traditional academic settings often isolate fields, making it hard to form interdisciplinary links.

CONCEPTUAL BRIDGE IDENTIFICATION

AI can recognize conceptual links across fields by analyzing:

Shared Vocabulary: When different fields use similar terminology, they may address related questions. AI can identify these overlaps even when fields don't typically interact.

Analogous Frameworks: Various fields may develop similar theories independently. Recognizing these similarities can promote fruitful cross-discussion.

Complementary Perspectives: Fields that examine similar phenomena from different viewpoints (e.g., economists and psychologists both studying decision-making) can benefit from integration.

METHODOLOGICAL TRANSFER OPPORTUNITIES

Methods created in one field often prove useful in others. AI can recognize:

Underutilized Methods: Techniques that are well-established in one area but are seldom used in related fields where they could be relevant.

Emerging Methods: New analytical or experimental approaches in their early adoption phase that could be applied to other fields.

Method Combinations: Opportunities to merge complementary techniques from various fields to answer questions neither could handle alone.

For example, network analysis methods from sociology have been applied in neuroscience, ecology, and organizational research.[17] AI can assist researchers in finding similar opportunities for methodological transfer.

COLLABORATIVE OPPORTUNITY IDENTIFICATION

Building effective interdisciplinary teams requires identifying researchers with complementary expertise who share an interest in specific questions. AI can help facilitate this by:

Expertise Mapping: Developing profiles of researchers' expertise based on publication records, grant awards, and stated interests.

Collaboration Network Analysis: Identifying researchers who have effectively worked across disciplines, highlighting possible partners for new initiatives.

Complementarity Assessment: Determining if specific researchers' expertise genuinely complements each other compared to redundant overlap.

Identifying Gaps in Teams: Recognizing when proposed teams lack essential expertise needed for interdisciplinary work.

PRACTICAL IMPLEMENTATION STRATEGIES

Effective AI use for research ideas needs careful planning and realistic expectations.

STARTING WITH QUESTIONS, NOT TOOLS

The biggest mistake is beginning with AI capabilities and looking for applications instead of starting with research challenges and investigating whether AI can assist. Successful implementation starts with clearly stating what you aim to achieve.

- What knowledge gaps concern you most?
- What trends do you need to understand?

- What stakeholder needs do you want to address?
- What feasibility questions do you face?

Only after clarifying these questions should you explore AI tools that might assist in answering them.

COMBINING AI WITH HUMAN JUDGMENT

AI should enhance, not substitute, human creativity and judgment in research ideation. Effective approaches include:

AI for Breadth: Using AI to analyze extensive literature, recognize patterns, and reveal possibilities you might not find otherwise.

Humans for Depth: Using domain expertise, critical thinking, and judgment to assess AI-generated opportunities and decide which ones are worth pursuing.

AI for Validation: Using AI to evaluate feasibility, analyze resources, and identify potential barriers for ideas generated through human creativity.

Humans for Prioritization: Making final decisions about research directions based on values, mission alignment, and strategic considerations that AI cannot assess.

ITERATIVE EXPLORATION

Research ideation seldom follows a straight path from question identification to a complete research plan. Instead, it involves repeated cycles of exploration, refinement, and redirection. AI tools should facilitate this iterative process.

- Initial broad scans to identify possibilities
- Focused deep dives on promising areas
- Feasibility checks that may redirect to related questions
- Stakeholder validation that may refine priorities
- Resource assessment that may adjust scope

AI allows more exploration cycles in less time, helping researchers find the best questions more efficiently.

MAINTAINING CRITICAL PERSPECTIVE

AI analysis of literature and trends reflects current research priorities and biases. Important questions may be understudied because they've been overlooked or undervalued. AI trained on existing literature can perpetuate these gaps.

RESEARCHERS SHOULD ASK

- Are there crucial questions that AI isn't highlighting because the research community has traditionally overlooked them?
- Do identified trends represent real scientific significance or just current fads?
- Whose perspectives and priorities are reflected in the data AI analyzes, and whose are absent?

Critical evaluation of AI-driven opportunities ensures research aligns with broader goals beyond merely following current trends.

Capabilities and Limitations: The Ideation Audit

While Chapter 1 establishes the broad capabilities of AI in Semantic Synthesis and Pattern Recognition, applying these to research ideation requires a specific set of Override Triggers. AI can effectively map the "known universe" of published data to identify gaps, but it cannot navigate the "unwritten realities" of clinical practice or institutional logistics (Table 2.1).

The Novelty Trap and "Hallucinated Feasibility"

A critical limitation in this phase is the Novelty Bias. Because LLMs are trained on existing patterns, truly revolutionary ideas, the "black swans" of science, often appear as statistical errors to the AI. As you use AI to brainstorm, you must apply the Adversarial Questioning protocol:

- **The AI Limit**: AI can show you what *is*; it struggles to imagine what *isn't*.

TABLE 2.1
Ideation-Specific Override Protocols

Ideation Task	AI Execution (The "Meat")	The Human Override (The Top Bread)
Gap analysis	Scanning thousands of papers to find "white space" or unstudied correlations	**Sanity Check:** Determine if the "gap" exists because it is a breakthrough opportunity or because it is biologically/ logistically impossible
Trend extrapolation	Forecasting future research directions based on patent filings and news	**Strategic Pivot:** AI identifies *consensus* trends; the human must identify *contrarian* opportunities that algorithms dismiss as noise
Hypothesis generation	Suggesting novel research questions and experimental frameworks	**Feasibility Audit:** Prune AI-generated plans to fit real-world resource constraints, clinical workflows, and patient burden
Cross-disciplinary links	Identifying connections between disparate fields (e.g., Immunology and Material Science)	**Value Judgment:** Decide if the link is scientifically significant or merely a statistical coincidence with no clinical utility

Refer to the Master Matrix in Section 1.3 for general failure modes; the table outlines the unique expert-level interventions required during the planning phase.

- **The Human Task**: You must provide the "Creative Leap." Use AI to organize the facts and then intentionally investigate the data points the AI suggests "discarding" as outliers.

Furthermore, even when AI successfully identifies a novel research avenue, it often suffers from Hallucinated Feasibility. It may propose methodologies that are statistically plausible but logistically or biologically impractical. For instance, recent simulations in cardiotoxicity research demonstrate that while AI can generate hypotheses with meaningful novelty, the resulting experimental designs are frequently overambitious and require significant human refinement to be executable.[14]

LOGISTICAL STRESS TESTING

AI-generated ideation lacks "grounding in the dirt." Before moving from an AI-assisted idea to a formal grant proposal (Chapter 3), the human investigator must trigger a **Logistical Stress Test** to account for variables the AI cannot "see":

1. **Staffing Reality**: AI ignores nursing ratios, clinician burnout, and the hours required for complex data entry.
2. **Patient Centricity**: AI may propose invasive procedures that ensure a 0% recruitment rate in a real-world clinical setting.
3. **Infrastructure Gaps**: AI cannot account for local supply chain delays, specific equipment backorders, or regional differences in Standard of Care.

The Override Trigger: If the AI suggests an experimental plan, the human must manually verify every "Execution" step against the current institutional resources. If the plan looks "perfect" on paper but impossible in the clinic, the Human–AI–Human Sandwich has failed at the top layer.

THE SKEPTIC'S CORNER

In the Human–AI Partnership, the greatest risk is automation bias, the tendency to accept AI output at face value. To counter this, researchers must treat AI as a hostile witness. Adversarial prompting is a deliberate strategy in which you command the AI to find flaws in its own reasoning, argue against your hypotheses, or act as a hypercritical peer reviewer. By forcing the AI to simulate a counterargument, you identify the weak points in your research before they reach a review board or a journal editor.

- **Target Task**: Identifying research gaps and novelty.
- **Adversarial Prompt**: "I am proposing a study on [Topic]. Identify three seminal papers I have likely overlooked and explain why my proposed research question might be considered incremental rather than transformative by a top-tier journal."

ETHICAL CONSIDERATIONS

Using AI for biomedical research ideation raises several ethical issues. These are based on the core ethical principles discussed in Chapter 1, especially the Belmont principles of respect for persons, beneficence, and justice as they relate to AI contexts.

BIAS AMPLIFICATION

If AI identifies opportunities based on existing literature and funding patterns, it might continue to reinforce historical biases in which questions are asked and by whom.[18] Researchers should actively consider:

- Are there underrepresented populations or perspectives in the data analyzed by AI?
- Do identified opportunities reinforce existing power structures or knowledge hierarchies?
- How can we guarantee that diverse voices influence research priorities?

PRIVACY AND CONSENT

Using AI to analyze patient forums, social media, or other public discussions to identify research needs raises questions about whether people posting expect their words to influence research priorities and whether this use respects their autonomy.

COMPETITIVE CONCERNS

If AI helps researchers uncover emerging opportunities, does this favor those with access to advanced tools, potentially increasing the gap between well-resourced and under-resourced institutions?

RESEARCH PRIORITIES

Should research priorities stem from algorithmic analysis of trends, or should they be guided by democratic processes involving diverse stakeholders? AI can inform but should not decide which questions matter.

LOOKING FORWARD

As AI capabilities keep developing, research ideation tools will probably become more advanced, easier to access, and better integrated into researchers' workflows.

Personalized opportunity feeds: Instead of generic literature alerts, AI can deliver highly tailored streams of relevant opportunities, trends, and connections based on each researcher's specific interests and skills.

Predictive Gap Identification: AI could move from recognizing current gaps to predicting future gaps, questions that will become crucial as knowledge progresses.

Collaborative AI Systems: Instead of individual researchers using AI tools separately, research teams may employ shared AI systems that aid in coordinating ideas among collaborators.

Integration with Research Design: AI for ideation can seamlessly connect with AI for biomedical research design, enabling researchers to transition smoothly from question identification to protocol development.

Autonomous Hypothesis Generation and Testing: Systems like Google's AI coscientist point to a future where AI agents can not only generate hypotheses but also refine them through simulated debate and critique, although human oversight of which hypotheses deserve real-world investigation will remain crucial.[15]

The goal is not to automate creativity but to broaden the range of possibilities researchers can explore, speed up the search for potential directions, and help make better decisions about where to allocate valuable research resources.

CONCLUSION

Research ideation, choosing which questions to pursue, may be the most important decision researchers make. AI cannot make these decisions, but it can greatly increase the information researchers consider when making them.

By processing extensive literature to identify gaps, analyzing trends to spot emerging opportunities, surfacing stakeholder needs that research can address, assessing the feasibility of potential projects, connecting researchers with relevant funding, and facilitating interdisciplinary collaborations, AI tools enable researchers to make more informed, strategic decisions about research directions.

The most effective approach combines AI's ability to process large volumes of data and recognize patterns with human strengths in creative synthesis, value judgment, and understanding context. Neither alone is enough; together, they can help ensure research resources are focused on questions that truly matter.

The next chapter examines how AI can help researchers secure funding for their research areas through improved grant writing and proposal development.

KEY TAKEAWAYS

- Research ideation involves identifying questions that are important, novel, and feasible, a challenging synthesis of various information sources.

- AI is effective at analyzing extensive literature to find gaps, contradictions, and underexplored areas.
- AI-driven trend analysis can assist researchers in identifying emerging fields and forecasting future opportunities.
- AI-enhanced stakeholder needs assessment ensures research targets real-world priorities.
- Feasibility analysis with AI offers data-driven estimates of resource needs and possible obstacles.
- Early empirical evidence indicates AI can generate research hypotheses with meaningful novelty, although experimental plans still need significant human refinement.
- Grant opportunity matching links researchers with appropriate funding through advanced analysis of funder priorities.
- Interdisciplinary opportunities arise through AI analysis of connections between concepts and methods across different fields.
- AI should enhance human creativity and judgment, not substitute it, the best strategy combines algorithmic scope with human insight.
- Critical evaluation ensures AI-generated opportunities align with broader research objectives beyond just following current trends.

QUESTIONS FOR REFLECTION

1. What research opportunities might you be missing because you can't fully process the relevant literature in your field and related disciplines?
2. How could analyzing stakeholder needs alter your research priorities or strategies?
3. What feasibility challenges do you encounter in potential research projects, and how could data-driven estimates assist you in planning more effectively?
4. Are there fields outside your own whose methods or ideas might relate to your research questions? How could you find these links?

5. How can you balance algorithmic analysis of research trends with independent thinking about which questions truly matter?
6. If AI can generate new research hypotheses, what is the researcher's unique contribution to the ideation process, and how should that contribution be recognized and credited?

NOTES

1. Bornmann, L., & Mutz, R. (2015). Growth rates of modern science: A bibliometric analysis based on the number of publications and cited references. *Journal of the Association for Information Science and Technology*, 66(11), 2215–2222. https://doi.org/10.1002/asi.23329. Note: Bornmann and Mutz reported varying growth rates depending on the metric used; the volume of cited references doubles approximately every 9 years, while the number of publications grows at a slower rate of roughly 3%–4% annually. Current estimates place global output above 3.4 million papers per year as of 2025.
2. Rossi, F. (Chair). (2025). AAAI 2025 presidential panel on the future of AI research. Association for the Advancement of Artificial Intelligence. https://aaai.org/about-aaai/presidential-panel-on-the-future-of-ai-research/
3. Rzhetsky, A., et al. (2015). Choosing experiments to accelerate collective discovery. *Proceedings of the National Academy of Sciences*, 112(47), 14569–14574. https://doi.org/10.1073/pnas.1509757112
4. For current AI tools supporting systematic literature analysis and gap identification, see Elicit (https://elicit.com), Semantic Scholar (https://www.semanticscholar.org), Scispace (https://typeset.io), and Rayyan (https://www.rayyan.ai). Tool capabilities and availability evolve rapidly; these represent the landscape as of early 2026.
5. Camerer, C. F. (2003). *Behavioral Game Theory: Experiments in Strategic Interaction*. Princeton University Press. https://press.princeton.edu/books/hardcover/9780691090399/behavioral-game-theory?srsltid=AfmBOoo4D8YjVR-D1Hq9CWYQdz1-X1ACK1CrG3aQgLtFg-QYktLSFhC7
6. Open Science Collaboration. (2015). Estimating the reproducibility of psychological science. *Science*, 349(6251), aac4716. https://doi.org/10.1126/science.aac4716

7. The reproducibility debate intensified in 2025 when a presidential executive order emphasized a "reproducibility crisis" in science, and the Paragon Health Institute recommended that the NIH devote at least $48 million annually to fund replication studies. See: Modern Sciences. (2025, July 28). Research replication can determine how well science is working. https://modernsciences.org/research-replication-methods-crisis-july-2025/; and Chemical & Engineering News. (2025, July 21). Amid White House claims of a research "replication crisis," scientists push back. https://cen.acs.org/research-integrity/reproducibility/Amid-White-House-claims-research/103/web/2025/06
8. Sever, R. (2025, March 11). Interview on life sciences preprint servers. STAT News. https://www.statnews.com/2025/03/11/life-sciences-preprint-servers-openrxiv-richard-sever-qa/. Note: About 14% of published biomedical research now exists first as preprints, with bioRxiv and medRxiv together drawing 10 million visitors per month.
9. openRxiv. (2025, December 30). openRxiv 2025 year in review. https://openrxiv.org/2025-year-in-review/. Note: As of the end of 2025, bioRxiv and medRxiv together host more than 389,000 preprints. BioRxiv alone posted 49,256 new manuscripts in 2025, its busiest year on record, with approximately 80% of manuscripts eventually published in peer-reviewed journals (average 250 days after preprint posting).
10. Doudna, J. A., & Charpentier, E. (2014). The new frontier of genome engineering with CRISPR-Cas9. *Science*, 346(6213), 1258096. https://doi.org/10.1126/science.1258096
11. Stuart, T., & Satija, R. (2019). Integrative single-cell analysis. *Nature Reviews Genetics*, 20(5), 257–272. https://doi.org/10.1038/s41576-019-0093-7
12. Bommasani, R., et al. (2021). On the opportunities and risks of foundation models. arXiv:2108.07258. https://arxiv.org/abs/2108.07258
13. Townsend, L., & Wallace, C. (2016). *Social Media Research: A Guide to Ethics*. University of Aberdeen. https://www.utwente.nl/en/bms/research/forms-and-downloads/socialmediaresearchethics.pdf
14. Sun, D., et al. (2025). AI-assisted hypothesis generation to address challenges in cardiotoxicity research: Simulation study using ChatGPT with GPT-4o. *Journal of Medical Internet Research*, 27, e66161. https://doi.org/10.2196/66161

15. Gottweis, J., et al. (2025). Towards an AI co-scientist. arXiv:2502.18864. https://arxiv.org/abs/2502.18864. See also: Google Research. (2025, February 18). Accelerating scientific breakthroughs with an AI co-scientist. https://research.google/blog/accelerating-scientific-breakthroughs-with-an-ai-co-scientist/. Note: The AI co-scientist uses a "generate, debate, and evolve" framework with specialized agents (Generation, Reflection, Ranking, Evolution, Proximity, and Meta-review) and was validated in wet-lab experiments for AML drug repurposing and liver fibrosis epigenetic targets.
16. West Virginia University Health Sciences. (2025). Be$tMatch: An AI tool to help faculty researchers find matching funding opportunities. https://medicine.hsc.wvu.edu/News/Story?headline=betmatch-ai-tool-to-help-faculty-researchers-find-matching-funding-opportunities
17. Barabási, A. L., et al. (2011). Network medicine: A network-based approach to human disease. *Nature Reviews Genetics*, 12(1), 56–68. https://doi.org/10.1038/nrg2918
18. Mehrabi, N., et al. (2021). A survey on bias and fairness in machine learning. *ACM Computing Surveys*, 54(6), 1–35. https://doi.org/10.1145/3457607

3 AI for Grant Writing and Funding

THE GRANT FUNDING CHALLENGE

Research funding remains highly competitive, and recent policy shifts have made it even harder to navigate. At the National Institutes of Health (NIH), success rates for R01-equivalent grants, the main awards that make up most of the agency's research funding, dropped sharply in fiscal year 2025. The number of investigators receiving these grants decreased from 7,720 in 2024 to just 5,885 in FY2025.[1] Early-stage investigators (ESIs), those within 10 years of their graduate degree, saw their success rate fall from 26% in 2024 to 19% in 2025, despite an 11% increase in applicants.[1] Established investigators experienced a similar decline, with rates dropping from 27% to 20%, while "at-risk" investigators, those at risk of losing all funding, saw rates fall from 24% to 17%.[1]

Much of the decline has been linked to a Trump administration policy requiring NIH to fund multiyear grants upfront in a single lump sum, which forces the agency to allocate large portions of its annual budget to existing awards, leaving less for new grants.[2] The NIH acknowledged in a February 2026 blog post that this policy "was expected to lead to fewer awards and support fewer researchers overall," though NIH Director Jay Bhattacharya testified to the Senate that the drop was "not because of the policy necessarily."[1] With the Senate declining to reverse the policy for 2026, applicants should not anticipate immediate relief; in fact, data from the Association of American Universities shows that NIH issued 66% fewer grant

 DOI 10.1201/9781003782995-5

awards in the first 5 months of FY2026 compared to the same period's average during FY2021.[3]

The National Science Foundation (NSF) shows a more detailed picture. After years of decreasing application numbers, NSF success rates had increased to 28% overall by 2020, with some directorates like biology reaching 36%.[4] However, success rates vary greatly among directorates, and the computing directorate, which now receives 20% more proposals than 10 years ago, has maintained a success rate of only 24%.[4] More recently, NSF's Mathematical and Physical Sciences directorate reported a 27% funding rate in FY2024, indicating that success rates have stayed in a similar range but still differ by field.[4]

This competitive landscape takes a significant toll on researchers' time and well-being. Writing a major grant proposal is one of the most time-consuming activities in academic life. Estimates for an NIH R01 application range from 30 to over 100 hours, depending on the project's complexity, the number of collaborators, and whether the application is new or a resubmission.[5] One study of Australian medical researchers found that a new research council proposal took an average of 38 working days, with resubmissions requiring 28 days.[6] Many researchers submit the same proposal multiple times, incorporating reviewer feedback across cycles, a process that can span years. The emotional toll of repeated rejections can be significant, especially for early-career investigators building their programs in an environment where fewer than one in five applications are successful.

The grant-writing process involves several interconnected tasks: identifying opportunities that match your research, framing your work to align with funder priorities, crafting a compelling story about its importance and feasibility, explaining complex science to reviewers who may not be specialists in your field, developing accurate budgets, ensuring compliance with formatting and content requirements, coordinating contributions from collaborators, and anticipating reviewer concerns. Many of these tasks require processing large amounts of information, recognizing patterns, and systematically applying rules, areas where artificial intelligence (AI) can help. However, the most crucial elements, such as vision, creativity, and judgment that make research fundable, remain inherently human.

PROPOSAL DRAFTING AND OPTIMIZATION

Writing grant proposals takes hundreds of hours from researchers. AI can assist in many ways while keeping the human voice and vision that make proposals compelling.

LITERATURE SYNTHESIS AND BACKGROUND DEVELOPMENT

Grant proposals need clear and brief summaries of existing knowledge that set the stage for the proposed work. AI systems can constantly track relevant literature and notify researchers about new publications that could inform their proposals, not through simple keyword matching but by recognizing conceptually related work even when terminology varies. More importantly, AI can create initial drafts of literature summaries by analyzing multiple papers and pulling out key findings, which researchers then refine and incorporate into their narratives. By outlining what existing research has covered and what it has missed, AI can also help researchers identify the knowledge gaps their proposed work aims to fill, an essential part of any strong proposal. Citation management tools with AI features can ensure references are accurate, properly formatted, and strategically chosen to show thorough knowledge of the field.

PRELIMINARY DATA PRESENTATION

Most grant applications require preliminary data showing that the proposed approach is feasible. AI can help by creating publication-quality visualizations with appropriate statistical annotations, highlighting the most compelling patterns in early findings, and demonstrating how these findings connect to the published literature. These features assist researchers in making the strongest possible case for feasibility without misrepresenting their data.

WRITING ASSISTANCE AND REFINEMENT

A growing ecosystem of AI tools now directly supports proposal writing. General-purpose large language models (LLMs) like ChatGPT can assist with brainstorming, outlining, drafting, and editing, while custom GPTs allow researchers to create specialized grant-writing assistants with instructions tailored to specific funders or mechanisms.[7] Purpose-built platforms have also emerged: Grant Assistant, trained on over 7,000 successful proposals, can analyze Requests For Proposals (RFPs) and generate tailored drafts that match funder tone and requirements, claiming to reduce writing time by up to 70%.[8] Instrumentl offers AI-powered RFP analysis that identifies priorities, eligibility details, and narrative expectations and then provides a structured outline with guided drafting suggestions based on funder language and historical giving data.[9] Grantable focuses on rapid narrative generation from uploaded RFPs.[7]

While these efficiency gains are significant, they vary based on task complexity and researcher expertise. Independent empirical research on high-level professional writing tasks suggests a more conservative, yet still transformative, baseline for these productivity claims. For instance, controlled studies have documented a 40% reduction in drafting time coupled with an 18% increase in output quality.[9] These "productivity lifts" are frequently more pronounced for repetitive administrative sections of a proposal, such as facilities descriptions or biosketch formatting, than for the core scientific rationale.[10]

These tools can genuinely assist with clarifying language (such as reducing jargon or overly complex sentences), ensuring consistency (like aligning terminology and timelines throughout the proposal), enhancing readability, and smoothing transitions between sections. However, they have a key limitation: AI-generated text often sounds generic and lacks the authentic researcher voice that engages reviewers. Seasoned reviewers can usually identify formulaic AI writing, and proposals that seem template-driven or "AI-heavy" rarely succeed in competitive contexts.

Following the Human–AI–Human Sandwich model, effective use involves AI supporting, rather than replacing, human writing. The most successful proposals use AI to generate first drafts of administrative or descriptive sections that researchers then significantly revise. This ensures that the primary scientific narrative remains rooted in the researcher's unique clinical perspective and authoritative voice.[11]

COMPLIANCE CHECKING

Grant applications must meet various formatting and content requirements that differ among funders. AI can add value here with minimal risk. AI tools can verify fonts, margins, page limits, and section organization meet funder specifications; confirm all required sections are included and address specific questions; ensure budget requests align with proposed activities and that timelines are consistent; and verify institution-specific documents and approvals are submitted. These mechanical checks help catch errors that could lead to desk rejection before scientific review even starts.

STRATEGIC FRAMING AND POSITIONING

How research is framed significantly influences funding success. AI can assist in strategic positioning by analyzing characteristics of previously funded projects from target programs to identify effective framing strategies, ensuring the proper inclusion of terminology used in successful proposals. It can also analyze funder strategic plans and funded project portfolios to understand what the funder truly values beyond stated objectives and map the competitive landscape to find opportunities for differentiation.

However, strategic positioning ultimately relies on human judgment about genuine alignment between research interests and funder priorities. AI may unintentionally encourage researchers to choose safe, incremental approaches that replicate past successes instead of pursuing bold proposals that break new ground. Misrepresenting research to match perceived funder interests is both unethical and usually ineffective; reviewers are experts who can easily detect when proposals lack sincerity.

BUDGET DEVELOPMENT AND JUSTIFICATION

Accurate, well-justified budgets are crucial for proposal success and are an area where data-driven AI support can be especially beneficial.

AI can analyze similar funded projects to provide data-driven cost estimates for personnel, equipment, supplies, travel, and other categories. By examining what comparable projects budgeted and how costs have evolved over time, AI helps researchers create realistic budget requests and identify areas where their proposals might be over- or underbudgeted compared to similar work. For multiyear projects, AI can apply appropriate inflation factors, ensure budget distribution across years aligns with proposed activity timelines, and link budget phases to project milestones.

Budget justification, which explains why each expense is necessary, is another area where AI can assist in creating useful initial drafts. AI can generate first versions based on proposal goals and methods, identify budget items that lack sufficient justification or are disconnected from proposed activities, and verify that requests align with proposed sample sizes, timelines, and techniques. As always, researchers need to review and refine these drafts to ensure they are accurate and detailed enough.

MATCHING RESEARCHERS TO FUNDING OPPORTUNITIES

The funding landscape is extensive and constantly changing, making it truly hard for researchers to find all relevant opportunities. This is one of the most developed areas of AI use in the grant ecosystem.

AI systems can now continuously monitor funding announcements from government agencies, private foundations, professional societies, industry sponsors, and international funding bodies and then match opportunities to individual researcher profiles. Be$tMatch, developed at West Virginia University, uses LLMs to analyze NIH Notices of Funding Opportunity and match them to faculty research profiles, delivering personalized notifications every 2 weeks.[12] Commercial platforms like Instrumentl offer similar capabilities across multiple funding databases.[13] These tools go beyond simple keyword matching: they analyze researcher publication histories, stated interests, institutional affiliations, and career stages to surface relevant opportunities that researchers might not discover through manual searching.

AI can also uncover lesser-known opportunities by analyzing agency budgets, strategic plans, and administrative documents and predict when new funding rounds may occur based on past patterns. For opportunities that require collaborations involving multiple investigators or institutions, AI can identify potential partners with complementary skills and track records, evaluate whether proposed teams have all necessary expertise, and indicate which funding mechanisms need specific types of partnerships.

When primary funding sources seem unlikely to succeed, AI can propose alternative options: private foundations aligned with the research, industry partners interested in the questions, international funding channels, or mechanisms tailored for early-career investigators.

UNDERSTANDING YOUR REVIEW AUDIENCE

Understanding who may review your proposal and what they value helps researchers frame their work effectively. AI can analyze reviewer assignment patterns for target programs, identify likely reviewers based on publication records and expertise, and evaluate the range of expertise usually present on relevant review panels.

This Information Serves Important Purposes: it aids researchers in deciding how much background to include, which terminology to choose, and which parts of their work to highlight. By examining reviewer comments on similar past proposals, AI can also assist researchers in predicting common criticisms, questions about feasibility, and concerns about impact, so they can address these issues proactively.

An Important Ethical Warning: the purpose of understanding your audience is to communicate more effectively, not to manipulate the review system. Using AI to leverage knowledge of individual reviewers' biases or preferences crosses an ethical line. The difference between customizing your message for your audience, something every effective writer does, and manipulating the review process must be clear.

SUCCESS PROBABILITY ANALYSIS

While funding success depends on many factors beyond proposal quality, AI can offer assessments that guide strategic decisions on where to focus proposal development efforts.

AI can evaluate proposal drafts by comparing them to characteristics of successful versus unsuccessful proposals, focusing on clarity, completeness, innovation indicators, and feasibility signals based on similar programs. These evaluations don't determine funding decisions; factors like reviewer makeup, competition in a cycle, and funder budgets all influence outcomes and are beyond AI's ability to assess, but they can help researchers identify areas for improvement before submitting.

For researchers planning multiple submissions, AI can guide portfolio strategy by balancing high-risk, high-reward proposals with more secure options, scheduling submissions to allow sufficient development time while maintaining a steady funding flow, and analyzing whether resubmitting to the same funder or seeking alternative sources is more strategic. AI can also evaluate funder fit by examining whether a proposal's budget, scope, and framing align with typical expectations for a particular mechanism, helping researchers decide whether to submit or look for better-matched alternatives.

POSTAWARD GRANT MANAGEMENT

Securing funding is just the start. Effective grant management is crucial for maintaining funder relationships and positioning for ongoing support.

AI can assist with ongoing grant management by monitoring progress against proposed timelines and alerting investigators when milestones are approaching or deadlines are at risk. It can also track spending against budgets to identify potential overruns or underspending and generate initial drafts of progress reports based on research outputs during the reporting period. For publication and output tracking, a standard reporting requirement, AI can monitor papers published that acknowledge the grant, track citations as evidence of impact, document conference presentations, and record student and trainee outcomes.

Grants come with compliance requirements that vary among funders, and AI can assist in managing these obligations: tracking investigator effort reports, monitoring institutional review board approval status and adverse event reports, ensuring financial expenditures adhere to funder rules and institutional policies, and flagging inventions or discoveries that might need intellectual property disclosure. When project circumstances change, AI can also help with rebudgeting analysis, assessing whether proposed changes are allowable under funder rules and preparing justifications, and with drafting no-cost extension requests.

ETHICAL CONSIDERATIONS AND RESPONSIBLE USE

Using AI for grant writing raises important ethical considerations that researchers must navigate carefully. These build on the foundational ethical principles discussed in Chapter 1, particularly transparency, accountability, and fairness.

AUTHENTICITY AND MISREPRESENTATION

The most fundamental concern is authenticity. Proposals represent commitments to do specific work, and they should reflect the researcher's genuine vision, voice, and capabilities. Submitting AI-generated text without significant human refinement risks creating proposals that don't truly represent the researcher, a problem that can surface during study section discussions when investigators can't speak fluently about their own proposals. AI assistance in writing should never lead researchers to propose work beyond their actual capabilities, and the underlying research concepts should come from researchers, not be taken from AI analysis of others' work.

FUNDER DISCLOSURE REQUIREMENTS

The regulatory landscape for AI use in grant preparation is changing quickly, and researchers need to stay updated. NIH issued guidance (NOT-OD-23-149) in June 2023 that specifically bans peer reviewers from using AI tools to evaluate grant applications, citing confidentiality breaches when content is uploaded to AI platforms.[14] NSF encourages researchers to disclose AI use in project descriptions while prohibiting reviewers from using nonapproved AI tools, as outlined in its 2025 Proposal and Award Policies and Procedures Guide.[14] The Foundation for Food & Agriculture Research released a comprehensive policy in November 2025 that explicitly bans AI in peer review.[15] As recently as March 2026, the American Diabetes Association introduced an AI policy that applies to all grant applications and peer-review processes.[16] These policies mainly target the review process, but disclosure requirements for applicants' use of AI in preparing proposals are expanding. Researchers should review current funder policies before each submission.

FAIRNESS AND ACCESS

If AI tools offer significant benefits in grant writing, unequal access to these tools could worsen existing disparities in research funding. Well-funded institutions might have access to premium AI platforms, dedicated grant support staff who can use AI effectively, and advanced computational infrastructure, advantages that deepen current inequalities.[17] Additionally, if AI learns from patterns in previously funded proposals, it could reinforce historical biases about what gets funded and who receives funding, systematically disadvantaging researchers from underrepresented groups or institutions.[14] Ensuring wider access to AI tools and carefully assessing AI recommendations for biases are crucial steps toward equity.

INTELLECTUAL PROPERTY AND CONFIDENTIALITY

Proposals include confidential information such as unpublished research ideas, proprietary methods, and preliminary data. When using AI tools, especially cloud-based services, it is essential to ensure that proposal content remains confidential and is not used to train AI models that could reveal your ideas to competitors. When AI assists in proposal development, concerns about intellectual property ownership may also arise, particularly with proprietary AI tools whose terms of service might claim rights over content processed through their systems.

CAPABILITIES AND LIMITATIONS: THE FUNDING AUDIT

While Chapter 1 establishes the broad capabilities of AI in Narrative Generation and Regulatory Mapping, applying these to grant writing requires a specialized set of Override Triggers. In the high-stakes environment of study sections and program officer reviews, AI can provide the structure, but only the human investigator can provide the Strategic Positioning and Authentic Voice required to win (Table 3.1).

TABLE 3.1
Grant-Specific Override Protocols

Grant Task	AI Execution (The "Meat")	The Human Override (The Top Bread)
Compliance checking	Screening the FOA/RFA for font, margin, and page limit requirements	**Final Audit:** Manually verify against the most recent NIH/NSF "Notice of Change" (NOT-OD) issued *after* the AI's training cutoff
Funder matching	Scanning databases (Dimensions, Grants.gov) against your research profile	**Relationship Check:** AI identifies *topics*; humans must identify *relationships*. Consult Program Officers to assess unstated priorities or current "political" climates

(*Continued*)

TABLE 3.1 (*Continued*)
Grant-Specific Override Protocols

Grant Task	AI Execution (The "Meat")	The Human Override (The Top Bread)
Budget justification	Drafting narratives based on line-item spreadsheets	**Cap Verification:** Manually verify salary caps and GSA per diem rates for 2026. AI often reverts to outdated fiscal year tables
Language refinement	Enhancing clarity and correcting grammatical flow	**Voice Restoration:** AI tends toward "neutral" prose. The PI must reinject the passion, urgency, and clinical "gravity" that engages human reviewers

Refer to the Master Matrix in Section 1.3 for general failure modes; the table outlines the unique expert-level interventions required for the funding phase.

THE "SAFE-BET" TRAP AND INNOVATION DILUTION

A significant risk in using AI for grant development is the Regression to the Mean. Because LLMs are trained on a vast corpus of "conventional" successful proposals, they inherently favor incremental science over bold, "high-risk, high-reward" innovation.

- **The AI Limit**: AI may unintentionally suggest "safe" research directions that align with past patterns but fail to excite a modern review panel looking for a "Paradigm Shift."
- **The Human Task**: You must intentionally protect the "Innovation" section of your proposal. If the AI suggests softening a contrarian hypothesis to make it more "plausible," this is a Red Flag that the AI is diluting your competitive edge.

STRATEGIC POSITIONING VERSUS PATTERN MATCHING

Winning a grant is as much about *where* the proposal sits in a funder's portfolio as it is about the science itself. AI can match keywords, but it cannot:

1. **Interpret "Between the Lines"**: AI cannot sense the shifting priorities of a new Institute Director or the "unspoken" preferences of a specific Study Section chair.
2. **Navigate Reputation**: Funding often depends on trust built over years of interaction. AI lacks the "institutional memory" of your specific department's track record.
3. **Manage the "Innovation-Diversity Paradox"**: While AI can audit for inclusive language, only a human can strategically balance the team's composition to meet specific agency goals for the 2026 fiscal year.

The Override Trigger: If the AI suggests a funding strategy or "Strategic Aim," the human must perform a Stakeholder Alignment Check. If the AI's suggested direction contradicts your recent conversations with a Program Officer, the AI output must be discarded. In grant writing, the AI is your *copyeditor*, but you remain the *Chief Strategist*.

THE SKEPTIC'S CORNER

- **Target Task**: Strategic framing and proposal drafting.
- **Adversarial Prompt**: "Now act as a highly skeptical NIH Study Section reviewer. Identify the three weakest links in my scientific rationale and list five specific reasons why you would score this proposal as 'low feasibility'."

PRACTICAL IMPLEMENTATION STRATEGIES

Starting Points

For researchers new to using AI in grant writing, the best approach is to start with specific, clearly defined tasks instead of trying to use AI for the entire proposal process. Tasks like literature synthesis, formatting checks, and budget benchmarking are low-risk starting points where AI output can be easily checked. As you gain experience, you can move on to drafting support and strategic analysis.

Throughout, three principles should guide your use: maintain control by using AI as a tool you direct rather than letting it drive content or direction; verify everything by never including AI-generated content without thoroughly checking for accuracy, appropriateness, and authenticity; and preserve your voice by extensively editing AI-generated text to ensure it reflects your genuine perspective and vision.

INTEGRATION INTO WORKFLOW

Effective AI use aligns with the natural stages of proposal development. In early exploration, use AI to scan funding landscapes and find opportunities. During mid-draft, employ AI for literature synthesis, initial section drafts, and organizing structure. In late refinement, apply AI for clarity checks, consistency verification, compliance review, and final formatting. After submission, analyze reviewer feedback with AI to detect patterns and improve future proposals.

TEAM COORDINATION

For multiinvestigator proposals, increasingly common in team science, AI can help ensure consistency across sections written by different team members, combine multiple perspectives into a clear narrative, and track changes made by contributors. These coordination tasks are tedious but important, and AI manages them effectively.

LOOKING FORWARD

The tools for AI-assisted grant writing will keep evolving quickly. Several new advancements are likely to change the field.

EVOLVING AI GRANT TOOLS

Real-time collaboration systems that support multiple investigators working simultaneously with smart integration will make team proposal development more efficient. More accurate predictive analytics based on proposal features, funder trends, and competitive environments will help researchers make better strategic choices. Personalized AI coaches that learn individual researchers' writing styles and areas for improvement will offer increasingly tailored support. And seamless integration between proposal development and postaward management platforms will lessen administrative burdens throughout the grant lifecycle.

REGULATORY AI ADOPTION AND ITS IMPLICATIONS FOR RESEARCHERS

AI is transforming not only how researchers write grants but also how funders and regulators process them. The FDA's launch of Enterprise Language Support Assistant (ELSA) in June 2025 highlights this trend.[18] ELSA is a LLM-powered tool deployed across the agency to help FDA staff read, write, summarize, and analyze regulatory documents. Developed within a high-security GovCloud environment, ELSA is already used to speed up clinical protocol reviews, reduce scientific evaluation timelines, and identify high-priority inspection targets.[18] By January 2026, the FDA expanded ELSA into full "agentic AI" mode, advancing from simple queries to multistep workflow planning.[19]

For researchers, ELSA's importance goes beyond the FDA. It reflects a larger trend: the agencies that review proposals, assess regulatory submissions, and oversee research compliance are themselves adopting AI. This has practical effects on how researchers prepare their submissions.

If AI-assisted reviewers can quickly cross-check claims against databases, identify inconsistencies, or highlight missing components, the standard for completeness and accuracy increases. Researchers should anticipate that the review process for funding will become more systematic and data-driven, even as human judgment remains essential for evaluating scientific merit.

Notably, ELSA's rollout has faced some challenges. In early 2026, the FDA was compelled to change ELSA's underlying model from Anthropic's Claude to Google's Gemini because of contractual shifts, a reminder that reliance on specific AI platforms can pose its own risks.[20]

However, the core of grant writing, crafting compelling visions for important research, will always be a human task that AI can assist with but not replace. The successful researchers will be those who leverage AI to manage the mechanical, analytical, and information-processing aspects of proposal development, while dedicating their own time to what matters most: developing innovative ideas, making convincing cases for their significance, and building the relationships and track records that make research fundable.

CONCLUSION

Securing research funding is crucial but increasingly challenging. NIH success rates have dropped to about one in five for most investigators, and policy updates indicate this trend will continue. AI presents real opportunities to improve the funding process by automating routine tasks, offering data-driven insights, aiding in proposal development, and simplifying grant management.

The most effective approach combines AI's strengths in data processing and pattern recognition with human strengths in creative vision, strategic thinking, and authentic communication. Used thoughtfully and ethically, with attention to funder disclosure requirements, equity concerns, and the need to maintain authenticity, AI for grant writing is not a shortcut but a tool that helps researchers navigate increasingly complex funding landscapes while staying focused on advancing knowledge through rigorous research.

The next chapter examines how AI can assist with the thorough literature review and knowledge synthesis that underpin both grant proposals and research implementation.

KEY TAKEAWAYS

- NIH grant success rates sharply declined in FY2025, with ESI rates dropping from 26% to 19%, emphasizing the importance of proposal efficiency and quality more than ever.
- A growing ecosystem of AI tools, ranging from general-purpose LLMs to specialized platforms like Instrumentl, Grant Assistant, and Grantable, supports proposal development from opportunity identification to postaward management.
- Literature synthesis, compliance checking, budget benchmarking, and funder matching are areas where AI provides significant, measurable value.
- AI cannot replace the authentic voice, strategic vision, and genuine commitment that make proposals fundable, experienced reviewers can often detect generic AI prose.
- Funder AI policies are evolving quickly: NIH bans AI in peer review, NSF mandates disclosure, and new policies from organizations like ADA keep emerging.
- Regulatory agencies are adopting AI (e.g., FDA's ELSA), which is changing how submissions are processed and increasing the standards for accuracy and completeness.
- Ethical use involves maintaining researcher authenticity, adhering to disclosure requirements, protecting confidential proposal content, and ensuring equity in AI tool access.

QUESTIONS FOR REFLECTION

1. How much time do you currently dedicate to grant-related activities, and which parts take up the most time?
2. Where in your grant-writing process could AI assistance be most helpful while maintaining your authentic voice and vision?
3. What concerns do you have about using AI for proposal development, and how could those concerns be addressed?

4. How could wider access to AI grant-writing tools impact equity in research funding?
5. What disclosure obligations do your target funders currently have regarding AI use in proposal preparation, and how will you stay updated as these policies evolve?
6. As funding agencies start using their own AI tools for review and evaluation, how could this alter the way you prepare submissions?

NOTES

1. Kaiser J. (2026, February 20). NIH research grant funding rates plummeted in 2025. *Science*. https://www.science.org/content/article/nih-research-grant-success-rates-plummeted-2025. Note: Data is for R01-equivalent grants. ESI success rates fell from 26% to 19%; established investigator rates from 27% to 20%; at-risk investigator rates from 24% to 17%.
2. Oza, A., & Wosen, J. (2025, December 18). NIH grant policy hurt funding chances for early-career scientists. https://www.statnews.com/2025/12/18/nih-early-career-researchers-grant-success-rate-falls/. Note: STAT reported that ESI success rates fell from 29.8% in FY2023 to 18.5% in FY2025, using a slightly different calculation methodology than NIH's February 2026 blog post.
3. Agarwal, K. (2026, March 19). Data show dramatic slowdown in NIH grantmaking. https://www.aau.edu/newsroom/leading-research-universities-report/data-show-dramatic-slowdown-nih-grantmaking. Note: NIH issued 66% fewer grant awards in the first 5 months of FY2026 compared to the same period's average during FY2021.
4. Mervins, J. (2022, May 9). Odds improve for winning NSF grants, but drop in applications troubles some observers. *Science*, 376(6594), 684. https://www.science.org/content/article/odds-improve-winning-nsf-grants-drop-applications-troubles-some-observers. Note: NSF success rates vary substantially across directorates, from 24% in computing to 36% in biology as of 2020. More recent data shows the Mathematical and Physical Sciences directorate reported a 27% funding rate in FY2024 (see https://www.nsf.gov/mps/funding-rates). Current rates across all directorates may differ; see https://www.nsf.gov/about/about-nsf-by-the-numbers for updated data.

5. Lee, K. (2025). 35 Grant Statistics for 2025: The Ultimate List. https://www.instrumentl.com/blog/grant-statistics-and-trends. Note: Estimates range from 15 to 20 hours for foundation grants to over 100 hours for complex federal proposals.
6. Herbert, D., et al. (2013). On the time spent preparing grant proposals: an observational study of Australian researchers. *BMJ Open*, 3(5), e002800. https://doi.org/10.1136/bmjopen-2013-002800. See also: https://researchwhisperer.org/2023/12/12/how-long-will-it-take-to-write-an-application/
7. Almeida, D. (2026, February 22). 7 AI grant writing tools tested on real NIH, NSF, and SBIR proposals: 2026 rankings. https://grantedai.com/blog/best-ai-grant-writing-tools-2026
8. FreeWill/Grant Assistant. (2025). The best AI grant writing tools for nonprofits in 2025. https://www.grantassistant.ai/resources/articles/the-best-ai-grant-writing-tools-for-nonprofits-in-2025. Note: Claimed 70% time reduction has not been independently validated in peer-reviewed research.
9. Noy, S., & Zhang, W. (2023). Experimental evidence on the productivity effects of generative artificial intelligence. *Science*, 381(6654), 187–192. https://doi.org/10.1126/science.adh2586
10. Brynjolfsson, E., Li, D., & Raymond, L. R. (2023). Generative AI at Work. *National Bureau of Economic Research (NBER) Working Paper No. 31161.* https://www.nber.org/papers/w31161. https://doi.org/10.3386/w31161
11. Dell'Acqua, F., et al. (2023). Navigating the Jagged Technological Frontier: Field Experimental Evidence of the Effects of AI on Knowledge Worker Productivity and Quality. Harvard Business School Technology & Operations Mgt. Unit Working Paper No. 24-013.
12. Carruthers, R. (2025). The best AI tools for grant writing in 2025: What nonprofits should know before choosing one. https://www.instrumentl.com/blog/best-ai-for-grant-writing
13. West Virginia University Health Sciences. (2025). Be$tMatch: An AI tool to help faculty researchers find matching funding opportunities. https://medicine.hsc.wvu.edu/News/Story?headline=be-tmatch-ai-tool-to-help-faculty-researchers-find-matching-funding-opportunities
14. Goldblatt, D. (2025). AI disclosure requirements in research and publishing. https://campus.kennesaw.edu/offices-services/research/ai-disclosure.php. Note: NIH NOT-OD-23-149 (June 2023) prohibits peer reviewers from using AI for grant analysis. NSF guidance formalized in 2025 PAPPG encourages applicant disclosure and prohibits reviewer use of nonapproved tools. DOD lacks specific research AI disclosure requirements.

15. Foundation for Food & Agriculture Research. (2025, November). Policy on prohibiting artificial intelligence tools in peer review. https://foundationfar.org/grants-funding/policy-on-prohibiting-artificial-intelligence-tools-in-peer-review/
16. American Diabetes Association. (2026, March 3). American diabetes association's policy on generative artificial intelligence use in research grant applications, Peer Review, and Reporting for Funded Awards. https://professional.diabetes.org/sites/dpro/files/2026-03/ada-Research-Programs-AI-Policy-for-Grants-3-3-26-FINAL.pdf
17. Mehrabi, N., et al. (2021). A survey on bias and fairness in machine learning. *ACM Computing Surveys*, 54(6), 1–35. https://doi.org/10.1145/3457607
18. U.S. Food and Drug Administration. (2025, June 2). FDA launches agency-wide AI tool to optimize performance for the American people. https://www.fda.gov/news-events/press-announcements/fda-launches-agency-wide-ai-tool-optimize-performance-american-people
19. U.S. Food and Drug Administration. (2026, January 11). FDA expands artificial intelligence capabilities with agentic AI deployment. https://www.fda.gov/news-events/press-announcements/fda-expands-artificial-intelligence-capabilities-agentic-ai-deployment
20. Chew, K., & Yang, M. (2026, March 11). FDA's Elsa AI switches from Claude to Gemini: What sponsors need to know. https://www.clinicalleader.com/doc/fda-s-elsa-ai-switches-from-claude-to-gemini-what-sponsors-need-to-know-0001

4 AI for Literature Review and Knowledge Synthesis

THE LITERATURE REVIEW CHALLENGE

The literature review is both important and challenging. Understanding existing knowledge is key to finding research gaps, avoiding duplication, contextualizing findings, and building on previous work. However, the volume of scientific literature has grown so much that a comprehensive review by individual researchers is nearly impossible.

The scale of the problem is massive. As explained in Chapter 1, over 3.4 million scientific papers are published each year across all fields.[1] PubMed alone, which mainly covers biomedical research, added about 1.57 million new citations in fiscal year 2023, and as of early 2026, it has over 40 million indexed citations, with 3.66 billion searches performed in FY2023.[2] Even within narrow specialties, researchers find it hard to stay updated with new publications. The problem isn't just the volume: relevant work may appear in unexpected places, use different terminology, or belong to related fields. Traditional keyword searches often miss conceptually related work that doesn't share the same words. As a result, important discoveries can stay hidden, undiscovered by those who could benefit most from them.

Beyond discovery, synthesis poses its own challenges. Finding relevant papers is just the beginning; extracting key details,

DOI 10.1201/9781003782995-6

identifying patterns across studies, reconciling conflicting findings, and integrating insights into coherent narratives require significant time and expertise. Literature review is not a one-time task; new publications continually emerge that may inform ongoing research, and staying up to date while conducting research is difficult but essential.

Quality assessment adds another layer of complexity. Not all published research is equally thorough or reliable, and evaluating study quality, identifying potential biases, and weighing evidence accurately require careful judgment and significant time. Perhaps most concerning is the growing challenge to integrity: the number of retracted papers has increased considerably, with 4,544 research papers retracted in 2025 alone,[3] yet retracted papers continue to be cited and influence research long after retraction notices are issued.[4] Identifying and removing problematic literature is essential for maintaining the integrity of the scientific record.

These challenges affect every aspect of research. Grant proposals require thorough literature reviews. Research design depends on understanding which methods have succeeded or failed. Data interpretation involves knowing how findings relate to existing evidence. Publishing involves placing new work within the broader literature. Traditional methods, such as manual database searches, reading abstracts and papers, taking notes, and synthesizing information, worked well when the literature was smaller, but they are increasingly struggling with the current volume and complexity. Artificial intelligence (AI) offers fundamentally new solutions to these challenges.

AI-POWERED SEARCH AND DISCOVERY TOOLS

The first step in a literature review is finding relevant work, and AI is transforming how researchers discover literature through semantic understanding, cross-database integration, and citation network analysis. A growing ecosystem of specialized tools now supports this process.

SEMANTIC SEARCH

Traditional database searches rely on keyword matching: papers are found only if they include the specific words searched for. AI-powered semantic search understands concepts and meanings, not just keywords, and this difference is crucial for thorough discovery.

Conceptual matching allows AI to identify papers on similar ideas even when different terms are used. A search for "machine learning" can bring up papers about "artificial intelligence," "neural networks," or "deep learning" based on conceptual links rather than exact word matches. Question-based search lets researchers ask questions in natural language, "What factors affect treatment adherence in diabetes patients?," and receive relevant results even if no paper contains that exact phrase. Example-based search goes further: researchers can provide a paper and ask for similar work, using AI's understanding of content, methods, and ideas to find related studies that traditional citation searches might miss.

Several tools now operationalize these capabilities. Semantic Scholar, developed by the Allen Institute for AI, indexes over 200 million papers and uses AI to extract key findings, identify methodological approaches, and highlight influential work.[5] Elicit specializes in evidence synthesis workflows, allowing researchers to ask natural language questions and receive structured answers drawn from the literature.[6] Consensus focuses specifically on extracting and synthesizing findings from peer-reviewed sources, making it especially useful for understanding what the evidence indicates about specific questions.[6] Undermind combines deep AI search with academic rigor, iteratively refining searches to surface highly relevant papers that traditional searches often miss.[7] Each tool has distinct strengths, researchers benefit from using multiple tools rather than relying on any single platform.

CROSS-DATABASE INTEGRATION

Scientific literature is stored across various databases, PubMed, Web of Science, Scopus, Google Scholar, and discipline-specific repositories, each with different interfaces, search conventions, and coverage. AI can unify these sources by searching multiple databases simultaneously, deduplicating results, identifying which databases are most likely to contain relevant work for specific queries, and, when possible, searching full text rather than just abstracts and titles. This integration is important because papers that don't mention key concepts in their abstracts might still contain significant findings hidden in methods or discussion sections.

CITATION NETWORK ANALYSIS

Understanding how papers relate through citations uncovers patterns not visible in traditional searches. Forward citation tracking shows all papers that cite a particular work, demonstrating how ideas are adopted, challenged, or expanded. Backward citation analysis examines which seminal works are cited by relevant papers, highlighting foundational literature. Cocitation analysis finds papers frequently cited together, indicating related or complementary work even if they do not directly cite each other.

Tools like Litmaps and Connected Papers visualize these citation networks graphically, making it easier to understand how research threads connect and where clusters of related work exist.[8] Scite goes further by analyzing citation context, understanding how papers are cited (supportively, critically, or as background) rather than simply counting citations.[9] This distinction matters: a paper cited 500 times primarily in critical contexts tells a very different story than one cited 500 times in support of its findings.

EMERGING LITERATURE DETECTION

AI can identify new research more quickly than traditional alert systems by monitoring preprint servers for relevant work months before peer review, tracking conference proceedings and presentations for early signs of emerging trends, and analyzing publication and citation rates to detect growing interest in topics. These early-warning capabilities give researchers the opportunity to engage with new findings before they become widespread.

AUTOMATED SUMMARIZATION AND EVIDENCE MAPPING

Once relevant papers are identified, efficiently extracting key information becomes crucial. AI helps with this through single-paper summarization, multipaper synthesis, and structured evidence mapping.

For individual papers, AI can generate concise summaries that highlight key findings, methods used, populations studied, acknowledged limitations, and novelty claims. These summaries help researchers quickly assess relevance and decide which papers warrant full reading. However, automated summaries should be viewed as screening tools rather than replacements for reading important papers in full; AI may miss nuances, mischaracterize findings, or fail to capture the significance of methodological choices.

Even more powerfully, AI can synthesize information from multiple papers, identify findings consistently reported across studies, flag contradictory results, recognize which methods are commonly used versus rare, show how understanding has evolved over time, and highlight questions frequently mentioned as needing research but not yet addressed. Chapter 2 discussed AI for identifying research gaps; the literature synthesis tools described here provide the raw material for that gap identification process.

For complex questions studied by many research efforts, AI can generate evidence maps that show what is well-established (areas with solid, consistent research), what remains uncertain (questions with limited or conflicting evidence), what is unknown (important questions lacking research), and how research focus is spread across subtopics. These maps assist researchers in positioning their own work and finding high-value opportunities.

AI can also systematically extract specific information from papers, such as sample sizes, demographics, intervention details, outcome measures, effect sizes with confidence intervals, and study quality indicators, enabling structured comparisons across studies and supporting meta-analyses. This ability transforms what would be weeks of manual data extraction into a process that can be completed in hours, although human verification of the extracted data remains essential.

RETRACTIONS, CORRECTIONS, AND RESEARCH INTEGRITY

The integrity of any literature review relies on identifying and properly handling retracted, corrected, or otherwise problematic publications. This presents both an increasing burden on the research community and an essential responsibility for ensuring scientific accuracy.

THE RETRACTION PROBLEM

Research retractions have grown significantly in recent decades, with the pace picking up. In 2025, there were 4,544 research papers retracted worldwide, with China responsible for about 40% and India 20%.[3] The Retraction Watch Database, which celebrated its 15th anniversary in 2025, now holds over 60,000 retraction records.[10] A large-scale Scopus study of 35,514 retracted publications from 2001 to 2024 found that data-related issues, involving accuracy, reliability, validity, and integrity, were the leading causes of retraction.[11]

The downstream effects are concerning. A detailed study of postretraction citation patterns revealed that retracted papers continue to be cited long after their retraction, and only about 5.4% of those citations acknowledge the retraction.[4] This indicates that, in most cases, readers of citing papers would not know that the original source had been retracted. The ripple effects spread through the scientific literature: researchers build on retracted findings, wasting time and resources on false leads; fields may spend years exploring directions based on fraudulent results; in medical research, retracted papers can influence clinical practices and potentially harm patients; and public trust in science diminishes with each high-profile retraction.

AI FOR RETRACTION DETECTION AND EXCLUSION

AI systems play a vital role in detecting and handling retracted literature. Automated retraction checks should be a core feature of any AI-enabled literature review tool, comparing papers with the Retraction Watch Database, PubMed retraction notices, and publisher-specific retraction lists. When retracted papers appear in search results or reference lists, AI systems should display clear warnings instead of considering them valid sources. Real-time monitoring should alert researchers when papers they cited or referenced are later retracted or corrected.

For systematic reviews and meta-analyses, AI must consistently exclude retracted papers from the evidence synthesis and document their removal. Citation network analysis can identify papers that heavily cite retracted work, alerting them for careful review as their conclusions may be affected. Moreover, AI should update continuously as new retractions happen, rather than only at the initial search.

THE RESPONSIBILITY FRAMEWORK

Multiple stakeholders share responsibility for addressing retractions, and the current system has notable gaps. Journals and publishers must clearly mark retracted papers, issue prominent retraction notices, maintain retracted papers with clear warnings instead of removing them entirely (to preserve the scientific record), and ensure retraction information spreads to all indexing databases.[12] Databases like PubMed, Web of Science, and Scopus must keep current retraction statuses, display clear warnings, and provide retraction details through Application Programming Interfaces (APIs) accessible to other tools. AI tool developers must incorporate retraction checks as a mandatory feature, refuse to include retracted papers in syntheses without explicit warnings, and document their retraction database sources and update frequency. Researchers must verify the retraction status of papers they cite, check for retractions both before and after manuscript submission, and correct their own work if they have cited papers that are later retracted.

CORRECTIONS AND EXPRESSIONS OF CONCERN

Beyond full retractions, papers can be corrected or flagged with expressions of concern. Corrections should be clearly indicated by AI systems, linking to correction notices so users know what has been changed. Expressions of concern are interim alerts when journals question the integrity of a paper but haven't confirmed misconduct; AI should prominently flag these papers and advise caution. Partial retractions, where specific figures, data, or conclusions are removed while the rest remains valid, require AI to clearly communicate which parts of the paper are still trustworthy.

PROACTIVE INTEGRITY CHECKING

Besides reacting to formal retractions, AI can actively support research integrity by detecting duplicate publications that may suggest redundant publishing or salami slicing, flagging papers with images that show signs of manipulation,[13] identifying statistical results that seem too good to be true or contain mathematical impossibilities, recognizing suspicious citation patterns that might indicate citation manipulation or paper mills, and checking for unusual author patterns. These proactive features help identify problematic papers before they require formal retraction, reducing the time during which flawed findings can affect other research.

SYSTEMATIC REVIEWS AND META-ANALYSES

Systematic reviews, thorough, organized literature reviews following clear protocols, are regarded as the highest form of evidence but are very labor-intensive. AI can assist with multiple parts of the systematic review process, and this is one of the most rapidly evolving areas of AI use in research.

SCREENING AND SELECTION

Systematic reviews often start with thousands of potentially relevant papers that need to be screened against inclusion criteria, a process that can take weeks of human effort. AI can handle title and abstract screening to identify papers that meet inclusion criteria while highlighting borderline cases for human review. Studies consistently show that AI-assisted screening can cut human screening time by 30%–50% while still maintaining high sensitivity for finding relevant papers.[14] Tools like Rayyan, originally created for systematic review screening, now include AI prioritization that learns from reviewer decisions to bring the most likely relevant papers to the top first.[15] Population Intervention Comparison Outcomes (PICO) Portal uses AI to speed up the screening process for clinical systematic reviews specifically.

Beyond screening, AI can more reliably identify duplicate records across databases than manual review, systematically verify retraction status, assist with full-text review by highlighting relevant sections and flagging potential reasons for inclusion or exclusion, and ensure screening decisions stay aligned with defined criteria.

DATA EXTRACTION AND QUALITY ASSESSMENT

Systematic reviews involve extracting specific data from included papers into structured formats, a tedious but essential task. AI can consistently extract designated data elements from papers across all studies, flag when papers fail to report expected information, and verify that the data extracted matches the source documents. For quality assessment, AI can determine whether studies meet set criteria, identify potential sources of bias based on study design and reporting, and assess reporting completeness against established guidelines such as Consolidated Standards of Reporting Tools (CONSORT) for randomized trials,[16] Preferred Reporting Items for Systematic Reviews and Meta-analyses (PRISMA) for systematic reviews,[17] and Strengthening and Reporting of Observational Studies in Epidemiology (STROBE) for observational studies.[18] However, ultimately, quality assessment requires human judgment on whether identified issues substantially impact study validity, a determination AI cannot reliably make.

META-ANALYSIS SUPPORT

When systematic reviews include quantitative synthesis, AI can help extract numerical results for analysis, evaluate statistical heterogeneity across studies, suggest potential moderators based on study features, and apply statistical methods to identify publication bias. These functions speed up the analysis process while preserving the statistical rigor required by meta-analyses.

THE COCHRANE INITIATIVE

In February 2026, Cochrane, the gold standard for systematic review methodology, launched a landmark study to assess whether AI tools can support or improve evidence synthesis.[19] Using an innovative adaptive platform study design, the initiative received 48 proposals from AI tool developers and, in March 2026, selected two tools for evaluation: Laser AI (developed by Evidence Prime) and Nested Knowledge. Testing will occur across about 15 Cochrane review updates, with results expected in the second half of 2026.[19] Cochrane explicitly noted that many existing evaluations of AI tools have methodological limitations and rely on studies conducted by tool developers, and that their study aims to bring independent, prospective, reproducible methods to this rapidly evolving field. This initiative indicates both the maturity and the remaining uncertainty of AI applications in systematic review; the tools are promising enough to merit rigorous independent evaluation, but the evidence base for their use is not yet conclusive.

LIVING LITERATURE REVIEWS

Traditional literature reviews are static snapshots, outdated as soon as completed. "Living literature reviews," continuously updated as new evidence emerges, have long been an aspiration, but AI makes them genuinely feasible.

AI can continuously monitor multiple databases, preprint servers, and publisher feeds for new publications, running predefined searches at regular intervals and alerting researchers when new relevant papers appear. When new studies are identified, AI can assess whether they meet inclusion criteria, evaluate quality, verify retraction status, and integrate findings into existing syntheses. Perhaps most valuably, AI can detect when new evidence substantially changes previous conclusions, flagging these shifts for human attention rather than requiring researchers to manually re-evaluate all new publications.

The result is a dynamic rather than static evidence summary: an always-updated synthesis that not only shows the current state of evidence but also how understanding has changed over time, where confidence is increasing or decreasing, what gaps remain, and whether any key papers have been retracted or corrected since the last review. Living reviews are especially useful in rapidly changing fields, for clinical guidelines that need frequent updates, and for ongoing research programs that require continuous awareness of the evidence landscape.

KNOWLEDGE GRAPH CONSTRUCTION

Knowledge graphs represent information as networks of entities, concepts, people, techniques, outcomes, and the relationships between them, enabling sophisticated analysis of knowledge structures that go beyond what traditional literature review can achieve.

AI can identify key entities in literature such as theoretical concepts, experimental methods, studied populations, tested interventions, and reported outcomes and recognize the relationships among them: causal links, methodological connections, temporal sequences, and contradictions. Once built, these graphs enable powerful analyses. Path finding can uncover connections between seemingly unrelated concepts through intermediary links. Centrality analysis highlights which concepts, methods, or researchers are most influential in the field. Cluster detection identifies groups of related work that may represent subdisciplines. Gap identification spots potential relationships that haven't been explored. Additionally, integrity tracking can trace how retracted papers have affected citation networks, revealing potentially compromised downstream research.

Knowledge graphs also support hypothesis generation by identifying missing links (plausible but uninvestigated relationships), recognizing patterns in one area that might apply to others through analogical reasoning, and suggesting explanations for inconsistencies across studies. These capabilities directly relate to the research ideation applications discussed in Chapter 2.

STAYING CURRENT IN YOUR FIELD

A literature review is an ongoing process, and AI allows for more advanced current awareness strategies than simple keyword alerts.

Intelligent alerting systems now offer concept-based notifications (for relevant papers regardless of specific terminology), priority-ranked results (ordered by predicted relevance instead of publication date), and surprise detection (highlighting papers that challenge conventional understanding). Retraction alerts provide instant notifications when papers you've cited are retracted or corrected. Over time, these systems learn individual researcher interests and refine their relevance assessments accordingly.

On a broader scale, AI can assist researchers in monitoring their field's landscape by identifying emerging topics, recognizing shifts in consensus or new controversies, tracking the adoption of innovative methods, and following the work of specific research groups. These capabilities are most effective when integrated into existing workflows, such as feeding information into reference managers, creating prioritized reading lists, annotating key passages in newly identified papers, and linking new publications to ongoing projects. AI should also automatically verify the retraction status of papers in reference libraries, offering a continuous integrity check that manual processes cannot provide.

CRITICAL READING AND INTERPRETATION SUPPORT

While AI can help identify and summarize literature, critical evaluation still requires human judgment. However, AI can support critical reading in important ways. For claim verification, AI can check that citations actually support the claims made about them and that cited papers haven't been retracted, verify that statistical claims follow from reported data, and spot inconsistencies between abstracts and full text or between different sections of papers. For assessing methodology, AI can recognize study designs and their implications, determine whether methods meet current best practices, and highlight potential concerns for human review. For context, AI can efficiently collect and present information about author expertise, funding sources, field reception of findings, and publication history, all of which inform critical interpretation but are time-consuming to gather manually.

QUALITY ASSESSMENT AND BIAS DETECTION

Not all published research is equally reliable, and AI can assist in quality assessment at various levels. AI can classify study designs (randomized controlled trials, cohort studies, case–control studies, and case series) and evaluate reporting quality based on established guidelines, CONSORT for randomized trials,[16] PRISMA for systematic reviews,[17] and STROBE for observational studies.[18] These automated checks can determine the proportion of recommended reporting elements present, offering a useful initial quality filter.

For risk-of-bias assessment, AI can flag indicators of selection bias, performance bias due to lack of blinding, detection bias in outcome assessment, attrition bias from differential dropout, and reporting bias from selective outcome reporting. AI can also identify signs of potential misconduct or paper mill origins, an increasingly important capability as the volume of fraudulent papers grows. However, nuanced quality judgment, determining whether identified issues genuinely threaten validity in the context of a specific research question, remains a fundamentally human task.

PRACTICAL IMPLEMENTATION STRATEGIES

Effective use of AI for literature review requires careful integration into research workflows rather than completely replacing existing practices.

STARTING WITH CLEAR QUESTIONS

A literature review should start with clear questions: What do I need to understand? What is the appropriate scope? What quality standards should I consider? How will I apply this information? Clear questions guide effective use of AI tools and help researchers determine whether AI-generated results meet their needs. A literature review supporting a grant proposal has different requirements than one for a systematic review or a clinical guideline, and the AI tools and methods should vary accordingly.

COMBINING AI WITH HUMAN EXPERTISE

The most effective literature reviews combine AI's strengths with human judgment in a deliberate partnership. AI offers breadth, scanning extensive databases and disciplines to find more relevant work than manual searches. Humans provide depth, applying expertise to evaluate important papers, assess quality, and make meaningful connections. AI increases efficiency, handling tasks like screening, data extraction, and summarization that take a lot of time. Humans focus on interpretation, understanding what findings mean, resolving contradictions, and recognizing implications. AI maintains integrity, systematically checking retraction status and spotting concerning patterns. Humans exercise ethical judgment, making decisions on handling borderline cases, conflicting evidence, or integrity issues.

VERIFICATION AND DOCUMENTATION

AI-generated literature reviews require thorough verification. Researchers should verify summaries against original papers, ensure retraction checking works properly, confirm that cited papers support the claims made about them, check for overlooked relevant work, and assess whether included papers meet quality standards. Keeping detailed documentation is also essential: recording search strategies (including AI tools used), screening criteria, retraction processes, quality assessment methods, and synthesis approaches allows others to evaluate the review's thoroughness and reproducibility.

ETHICAL CONSIDERATIONS

Using AI for literature reviews raises several ethical considerations that researchers must carefully navigate.

AI search algorithms might favor certain types of papers or sources, which could introduce systematic bias into reviews. Most AI tools function better with English-language papers, risking the exclusion of relevant work published in other languages, a significant issue for global research questions. AI cannot fix fundamental publication bias (where negative results are less likely to be published), but it can help identify its presence through statistical methods. Different databases have varying coverage; relying only on limited databases, even with AI help, may cause important work to be missed.

Transparency obligations require researchers to disclose when AI tools are used for literature review and clarify their role, enabling readers to evaluate potential limitations. Researchers are still responsible for accuracy even when using AI assistance; AI tools do not transfer this responsibility. Citation accuracy must be maintained whether references are assembled manually or with AI help, and vigilance for retractions should continue even after the initial review.

Equity issues also emerge: disparities in access to advanced AI literature review tools could worsen existing inequalities in research capacity. AI tools are only as good as the databases they can access, and paywalls and access restrictions limit AI usefulness for researchers at less-funded institutions. Making sure that retraction information is freely available to all AI tools and researchers is especially important for maintaining integrity across the research community.

CAPABILITIES AND LIMITATIONS: THE KNOWLEDGE SYNTHESIS AUDIT

While Chapter 1 establishes the broad capabilities of AI in Semantic Synthesis and Citation Assembly, applying these to a literature review requires the most rigorous Override Protocols in the research process. As documented in the Preface of this volume, AI-generated literature summaries are "conceptually sound" but "factually fragile." Without a human-led audit, the risk of propagating "hallucinated science" is a near-certainty (Table 4.1).

TABLE 4.1
Literature-Specific Override Protocols

Synthesis Task	AI Execution (The "Meat")	The Human Override (The Top Bread)
Broad discovery	Screening thousands of abstracts across disparate databases (PubMed, ArXiv, etc.)	**Relevance Audit:** AI identifies *keywords*; humans must identify *utility*. Manually vet the top 10% for methodological rigor before inclusion
Terminology bridging	Mapping how different fields (e.g., Immunology versus Engineering) describe the same concept	**Concept Validation:** Ensure the AI hasn't conflated two similar-sounding but biologically distinct mechanisms
Citation mapping	Tracking "seed" papers to identify key works and shifts in a research field	**Integrity Check:** Manually verify the retraction status of key works. AI often cites retracted "landmark" papers if they remain in its training data
Reference assembly	Generating bibliographies and in-text citations	**The 1:1 Audit:** As proven in this book's audit, 25% of AI citations are flawed. **Mandatory:** Every DOI and author list must be manually verified

Refer to the Master Matrix in Chapter 1, Table 1.1 for general failure modes; the table outlines the unique expert-level interventions required for knowledge synthesis.

THE PARADIGM BLIND SPOT

A critical limitation in AI-led synthesis is the **Consensus Bias**. AI models are trained on the "majority view" of existing literature. Consequently, they struggle to identify paradigm-shifting contributions, the "outlier" papers that fundamentally change a field, because these works often contradict the patterns the AI was trained to recognize.

- **The AI Limit**: AI can summarize what the field *thinks* it knows; it cannot recognize when the field is *wrong.*
- **The Human Task**: You must provide the "Critical Appraisal." Use AI to find the consensus and then intentionally look for the dissenting voices and methodologically superior (but perhaps less-cited) studies that the AI might deprioritize.

REAL SYNTHESIS VERSUS ALGORITHMIC SUMMARIZATION

True synthesis requires recognizing tensions, contradictions, and gaps, a task that depends on human analytical reasoning. AI can summarize a paper's abstract, but it cannot:

1. **Differentiate Quality**: AI often treats a poorly powered pilot study and a massive Phase III trial with equal weight if their abstracts use similar "impact" language.
2. **Detect "Hidden" Gaps**: AI identifies gaps based on what hasn't been *written.* Humans identify gaps based on what hasn't been *proven* in clinical practice.
3. **Contextual Importance**: AI cannot decide which among 5,000 papers "truly matters" for your specific clinical question. It lacks the "Professional Intuition" to prioritize a 10-year-old study that is suddenly relevant due to a new 2026 technological breakthrough.

The Override Trigger: If an AI summary claims "no evidence exists" for a phenomenon or provides a citation you do not recognize, you must trigger an Adversarial Search. Manually search for the specific counterevidence the AI might have missed due to its inherent preference for consensus data. In the literature review, the AI is your *librarian*, but you are the *Chief Scientist.*

THE SKEPTIC'S CORNER

- **Target Task**: Automated summarization and evidence mapping.

- **Adversarial Prompt**: "You just synthesized ten papers on [Topic]. Now, find two major contradictions between these studies that your summary smoothed over, and identify any cited authors who have recently had unrelated work retracted."

LOOKING FORWARD

AI capabilities for literature review continue to advance rapidly. Natural language models with a deeper understanding of scientific concepts and reasoning will enhance summarization and synthesis quality. Multimodal analysis, AI that can process figures, tables, and supplementary materials as effectively as text, will unlock information currently inaccessible to text-based tools. Real-time synthesis capabilities will make living literature reviews standard practice rather than just an aspiration. Predictive capabilities may eventually help researchers identify which papers are most likely to be influential or which findings are most likely to replicate. Improved integrity tools will provide more sophisticated detection of manipulation, fabrication, and paper mill outputs.

The Cochrane AI initiative marks a key milestone: an independent, thorough evaluation of whether AI tools can meet the high standards needed for top-quality evidence synthesis. With Laser AI and Nested Knowledge now chosen for testing in about 15 Cochrane review updates, results expected in the second half of 2026 will likely influence best practices for AI-assisted systematic reviews across fields.[19]

Seamless integration of literature review with writing, data analysis, and other research activities will lessen the difficulty of shifting between discovery and application. However, the fundamental nature of literature review, critically evaluating evidence to inform understanding, will still be mainly human work that AI supports rather than replaces.

CONCLUSION

A literature review is essential to research, but the rapid increase in scientific publications has made thorough reviews more difficult. AI provides powerful tools to tackle these issues, allowing for more comprehensive searches, more efficient screening and data extraction, systematic synthesis, and better staying current with new research.

Critically, AI systems have vital responsibilities for safeguarding research integrity by identifying and removing retracted publications, monitoring for corrections and expressions of concern, and helping recognize patterns that suggest misconduct. With over 4,500 papers retracted in 2025 alone and most postretraction citations failing to acknowledge the retraction, AI's role in maintaining the integrity of literature reviews is not just helpful; it is essential. Journals, databases, AI developers, and researchers all share the responsibility to ensure that flawed or fraudulent research does not continue to spread through the literature.

The most effective approach combines AI's capabilities in large-scale data processing, pattern recognition, and systematic quality checks with human strengths in critical thinking, contextual understanding, and nuanced judgment. AI can assist researchers in engaging more thoroughly with literature while ensuring the quality and integrity necessary for developing reliable knowledge.

The next chapter examines how AI can assist with hypothesis generation and research design, building on a thorough literature review to identify promising research directions and improve study methods.

KEY TAKEAWAYS

- Scientific literature has expanded beyond manual review capacity, with over 3.4 million papers published each year and PubMed now surpassing 40 million total citations.
- AI tools like Elicit, Semantic Scholar, Consensus, and Undermind enable semantic search, cross-database integration, and citation network analysis that surface relevant work much more effectively than keyword-based approaches.
- Automated summarization and synthesis assist researchers in efficiently processing large volumes of literature, although critical evaluation of key papers still requires human reading.

- Over 4,500 papers were retracted in 2025, and the Retraction Watch Database now contains over 60,000 records. AI systematically identifies and excludes retracted papers, safeguarding research integrity.
- Journals, databases, AI tools, and researchers all share responsibilities for properly managing retractions; most postretraction citations fail to recognize the retraction.
- Living literature reviews that continuously update as new evidence emerges become genuinely feasible with AI support.
- Cochrane's 2026 initiative, now testing Laser AI and Nested Knowledge across 15 review updates, will establish important benchmarks for AI-assisted evidence synthesis.
- Knowledge graphs facilitate advanced analysis of conceptual connections and aid hypothesis development.
- Quality assessment, bias detection, and critical interpretation still depend on human expertise and judgment.
- An effective literature review combines AI's processing power and integrity checking with human critical thinking and domain knowledge.

QUESTIONS FOR REFLECTION

1. How thorough is your current literature review process, and where could AI assist you in engaging more extensively with relevant research?
2. Have you checked the retraction status of the papers you regularly cite? How can AI tools assist in maintaining this watchfulness?
3. What role should AI tools have in systematic reviews and meta-analyses in your field, and how would you assess their reliability?
4. How might living literature reviews that continuously update change the way research is conducted and communicated?
5. What ethical responsibilities do researchers have in verifying AI-generated literature syntheses?

6. Which AI literature review tools are most useful for your specific research needs, and how will you verify their outputs?

NOTES

1. See Chapter 1, Note 1: Bornmann, L., & Mutz, R. (2015). Growth rates of modern science: A bibliometric analysis based on the number of publications and cited references. *Journal of the Association for Information Science and Technology*, 66(11), 2215–2222. https://doi.org/10.1002/asi.23329. Current estimates place global output above 3.4 million papers per year.
2. U.S. National Library of Medicine. (2024). MEDLINE PubMed production statistics. https://www.nlm.nih.gov/bsd/medline_pubmed_production_stats.html. Note: FY2023 data shows 1,567,478 new PubMed citations and 3.66 billion searches. PubMed now comprises more than 40 million cumulative citations as of early 2026.
3. Dr. Sunny. (2026, January 4). 4,500+ research papers were retracted in 2025: Countries, journals, and causes. https://phdtalks.org/2026/01/4500-research-papers-were-retracted-in-2025.html. Note: Data compiled from RetractionDatabase.org. China accounted for approximately 40% of retractions, India 20%.
4. Postretraction citation studies have consistently found that the vast majority of citations to retracted papers fail to acknowledge the retraction. One analysis found that only about 5.4% of postretraction citations acknowledged the retraction status. See: Wang, P., et al. (2023). Rising of retracted research works and challenges in information systems: Need new features for information retrieval and interactions. *Proceedings of the ACM Web Conference 2023.* https://dl.acm.org/doi/fullHtml/10.1145/3576840.3578281 (citing Teixeira da Silva & Vuong, 2022, among others). See also: Steen, R. G., Casadevall, A., & Fang, F. C. (2013). Why has the number of scientific retractions increased? *PLoS One*, 8(7), e68397. https://doi.org/10.1371/journal.pone.0068397
5. Semantic Scholar. Allen institute for AI. https://www.semanticscholar.org/. Note: Indexes over 200 million papers with AI-extracted key findings and citation context.
6. For current AI literature review tools, see Elicit (https://elicit.com), Consensus (https://consensus.app), and Scispace (https://typeset.io). Tool capabilities evolve rapidly; these represent the landscape as of early 2026.

7. Undermind. https://www.undermind.ai/. Undermind combines iterative AI search refinement with academic rigor. See community discussion: r/PhdProductivity. (2026, February). Tools for literature review in 2026.
8. Litmaps (https://www.litmaps.com) and Connected Papers (https://www.connectedpapers.com) provide visual citation network mapping. Both tools generate interactive graphs showing how papers relate through citation and conceptual similarity.
9. Scite. https://scite.ai/. Note: Scite analyzes citation contexts to classify how papers are cited, supportively, critically, or as background, providing a more nuanced picture than citation counts alone.
10. Retraction Watch. (2025, December 30). Cheers to 2025: In which Retraction Watch turned 15, and The Center For Scientific Integrity really became a center. https://retractionwatch.com/2025/12/30/cheers-2025-retraction-watch-turned-15-center-for-scientific-integrity/. Note: The Retraction Watch Database now includes over 60,000 retraction records.
11. Lendvai, G. F., & Sasvári, P. 'Wasted' research and lost citations: A scientometric assessment of retracted documents in Scopus between 2001 and 2024 (2001–2024). *Journal of Information Science*, 2025. https://journals.sagepub.com/doi/abs/10.1177/01655515251362383. Note: Analysis of 35,514 retracted publications found data-related problems (issues of accuracy, reliability, validity, and integrity) to be the dominant category of retraction causes. Readers are encouraged to consult the full text for detailed breakdowns by year and journal quartile.
12. Committee on Publication Ethics (COPE). (2019). Retraction Guidelines. https://publicationethics.org/retraction-guidelines
13. Bik, E. M., Casadevall, A., & Fang, F. C. (2016). The prevalence of inappropriate image duplication in biomedical research publications. *mBio*, 7(3), e00809–16. https://doi.org/10.1128/mBio.00809-16
14. Gates, A., et al. (2018). Technology-assisted title and abstract screening for systematic reviews: a retrospective evaluation of the Abstrackr machine learning tool. *Systematic Reviews*, 7(1), 45. https://doi.org/10.1186/s13643-018-0707-8. Note: While Abstrackr has been largely superseded by newer tools, the 30%–50% time reduction finding has been replicated across multiple platforms. See also: O'Connor, A. M., et al. (2019). Still moving toward automation of the systematic review process: a summary of discussions at the third meeting of the International Collaboration for Automation of Systematic Reviews (ICASR). *Systematic Reviews*, 8(1), 57. https://doi.org/10.1186/s13643-019-0975-y

15. Rayyan. https://www.rayyan.ai/. Note: Rayyan incorporates AI-assisted screening that learns from reviewer decisions to prioritize potentially relevant papers.
16. Schulz, K. F., et al. (2010). CONSORT 2010 Statement: Updated guidelines for reporting parallel group randomised trials. *The BMJ*, 340, c332. https://doi.org/10.1136/bmj.c332
17. Page, M. J., et al. (2021). The PRISMA 2020 statement: An updated guideline for reporting systematic reviews. *The BMJ*, 372, n71. https://doi.org/10.1136/bmj.n71
18. von Elm, E., et al. (2007). The strengthening the reporting of observational studies in epidemiology (STROBE) statement: Guidelines for reporting observational studies. *Lancet*, 370(9596), 1453–1457. https://doi.org/10.1016/S0140-6736(07)61602-X
19. Powell, M. (2026, February 18). Cochrane launches innovative study to assess AI tools for evidence synthesis. https://www.cochrane.org/about-us/news/cochrane-launches-innovative-study-assess-ai-tools-evidence-synthesis. See also: Cochrane. (2026, March 16). Cochrane announces selected AI tools for innovative platform study. https://www.cochrane.org/about-us/news/cochrane-announces-selected-ai-tools-innovative-platform-study. Note: Laser AI (Evidence Prime) and Nested Knowledge were selected from 48 proposals. Testing across ~15 Cochrane review updates is expected to conclude in the second half of 2026.

5 AI for Hypothesis Generation and Research Design

THE CHALLENGE OF HYPOTHESIS GENERATION AND RESEARCH DESIGN

Between identifying a research question and collecting data lies a vital step that decides whether a study will succeed: creating testable hypotheses and designing studies to evaluate them thoroughly. This phase requires a unique mix of creativity, technical skill, and careful judgment about methodological tradeoffs, and it is here that many research projects quietly succeed or fail.

The challenge starts with generating hypotheses. Moving from a broad research question to a specific, testable hypothesis involves recognizing patterns in existing data, identifying causal mechanisms that might explain observed phenomena, and creating predictions precise enough to be tested empirically. A good hypothesis falls between the obvious and the speculative: it needs to be new enough to add to knowledge but solid enough to test with available methods. Experienced researchers develop a sense for this balance over years, but even seasoned investigators can miss subtle patterns in large, complex datasets or overlook connections across different fields.

Once a hypothesis takes shape, complexity grows. Research design involves a series of interconnected decisions: what to measure, how to measure it, whom to study, how many participants to recruit, how to assign them to conditions, which covariates to control, what analyses to perform, and how to address inevitable issues like missing data, protocol deviations, and unexpected results. Each choice impacts the study's validity, feasibility, cost,

DOI 10.1201/9781003782995-7

and ethical considerations, and these impacts interact in complex ways that are hard to predict. A decision that maximizes statistical power might increase participants' burden; a design that ensures strong internal validity could limit its external validity for real-world use; a rigorous protocol might be impossible within budget and timeline limits.

These tradeoffs have traditionally been handled through researcher training, experience, and consultation with methodological experts, resources that remain crucial. However, artificial intelligence (AI) now provides truly new capabilities: the ability to explore extensive design spaces systematically, simulate study performance under different assumptions before data collection begins, and detect patterns in existing data that suggests hypotheses no individual researcher would have thought of. This chapter explores where these capabilities provide real benefit and where human judgment still remains indispensable.

PATTERN RECOGNITION IN EXISTING DATA

One of the most effective ways to generate hypotheses is by spotting unexpected patterns in data originally collected for other reasons. Large datasets, electronic health records (EHRs), population surveys, multiomics repositories, and administrative databases hold immense untapped potential for creating new research questions. The main challenge has always been the enormous scale: no human researcher can systematically examine all possible variable relationships in a dataset with thousands of features. AI transforms this challenge fundamentally.

SECONDARY DATA ANALYSIS FOR HYPOTHESIS GENERATION

Machine learning algorithms can systematically analyze large datasets to find associations that weren't part of the original research questions. A common example in biomedical research is drug repurposing: analyzing EHRs might show that patients taking a medication for one condition have unexpectedly lower rates of a seemingly unrelated disease, suggesting that the drug may have off-target therapeutic effects worth exploring further. This method has already led to real clinical insights, for example, AI-driven analysis of insurance claims and EHR data have pinpointed candidate drugs for repurposing against diseases ranging from Alzheimer's to certain cancers.[1]

Beyond simple associations, AI can identify more subtle patterns. Subgroup analyses can uncover different effects in specific populations that disappear in overall analyses; a treatment that seems ineffective on average could be highly effective in a particular demographic or genetic subgroup. Temporal pattern analysis can detect sequences and trajectories in longitudinal data that suggests causal mechanisms: does a change in a specific biomarker precede symptom onset by months, indicating a potential diagnostic or preventive opportunity? Dose-response mapping can determine the functional form of exposure–outcome relationships, helping to refine hypotheses about biological mechanisms. These capabilities don't replace the need for domain expertise; understanding why a pattern might occur is crucial for deciding whether it's worth exploring, but they greatly expand the range of patterns researchers can investigate.

CROSS-DATASET PATTERN RECOGNITION

Integrating information from multiple datasets can uncover patterns that are hidden within any single source. Meta-analytic pattern detection combines findings across studies to identify moderators: under what conditions a relationship exists and when it does not. In biomedical research, multiomics integration, combining genomic, proteomic, metabolomic, and phenotypic data, can map biological pathways and reveal markers linked to disease states or treatment responses in ways that no single data type alone could uncover.[2]Cross-context comparison helps determine whether patterns observed in one population, setting, or time period are replicated elsewhere, distinguishing reliable relationships from artifacts specific to certain contexts.

AI also supports the mechanical aspects of exploratory analysis that come before hypothesis formation. Automated visualization can produce various representations of data relationships, helping researchers identify patterns worth exploring. Anomaly detection can spot outliers that indicate genuinely interesting phenomena rather than just data errors. Dimensionality reduction techniques like t-distributed stochastic neighbor embedding (t-SNE) and uniform manifold approximation and projection (UMAP) help researchers find meaningful structure in high-dimensional data, revealing clusters or gradients that suggest underlying biological or behavioral groups.[3]

IMPORTANT CAVEATS

Pattern recognition in existing data generates hypotheses; it does not test them. This distinction is critical and ignoring it has contributed to the reproducibility issues discussed in Chapter 2. When AI analyzes thousands of potential relationships, some statistically significant patterns may arise by chance; these need prospective testing in independent samples before being considered confirmed findings. Patterns in observational data might reflect confounding factors rather than causation: the apparent link between a medication and lower disease rates could be due to differences between the patients who receive that medication and those who do not. Machine learning models can overfit to quirks of specific datasets, resulting in patterns that do not generalize. And statistical patterns, no matter how strong, do not reveal mechanisms; turning a pattern into a meaningful hypothesis requires human reasoning about why a relationship could exist, which remains a human contribution.

AI-GENERATED HYPOTHESES: EARLY EVIDENCE

The question of whether AI can generate genuinely useful research hypotheses has advanced from speculation to empirical testing. As discussed in Chapter 2, a 2025 study in the *Journal of Medical Internet Research* tested GPT-4o's ability to produce hypotheses for cardiotoxicity research, finding that 14% were rated highly novel and 65% moderately novel by expert evaluators, with existing literature found for only 29% of them.[4] Google's AI coscientist, introduced in early 2025, adopts a more structured approach using specialized agents that iteratively generate, debate, and refine hypotheses in a tournament-style framework.[5]

However, the most rigorous test to date, a large-scale study published in Science in August 2025, offers a more nuanced picture.[6] Researchers compared AI-generated scientific hypotheses with human-generated ones by having both evaluated blindly and then tested experimentally. The AI-generated hypotheses proved meaningful and testable, but they consistently lagged behind human hypotheses in novelty and experimental success when tested in real-world scenarios. The gap was not large, and the researchers noted it may be shrinking, but the finding emphasizes that hypothesis generation remains a domain where human scientific intuition still holds a significant advantage, at least for now.[6]

These results suggest the most effective approach is collaborative: using AI to generate a wide initial set of hypotheses that broaden the scope researchers consider and then applying human expertise to evaluate, refine, and prioritize the most promising candidates for further investigation. AI is good at providing breadth; humans are better at the judgment needed to identify promising leads from statistical illusions.

PREDICTING RESEARCH DIRECTIONS

Beyond analyzing existing datasets, AI can assist researchers in identifying promising opportunities by examining the structure and direction of the research enterprise itself.

CITATION AND PUBLICATION NETWORK ANALYSIS

The network of citations linking research papers encodes information about how fields develop. AI analysis of these networks can spot emerging connections, concepts, or methods that are starting to appear together but have not yet been widely studied, representing potential frontiers. It can also uncover underdeveloped areas where topics are often mentioned as needing investigation but remain empirically unexplored, cross-disciplinary opportunities where different fields approach similar questions with different frameworks, and declining research areas that might indicate either solved problems or prematurely abandoned directions that deserve reconsideration. These analyses complement the trend-analysis capabilities discussed in Chapter 2, but with a specific focus on identifying concrete, hypothesis-generating opportunities rather than broad thematic directions.

FUNDING AND TECHNOLOGY SIGNALS

Funding sources often predict future research trends, and AI can analyze grant databases to identify emerging priorities within funding agencies before they become widely recognized. It can also spot important questions that aren't currently receiving funding attention, potentially offering opportunities for researchers who can make compelling cases. Additionally, the rise of new technologies and methods creates further research opportunities. AI can monitor when measurement tools, experimental techniques, or analytical methods reach a level of maturity suitable for broader adoption, signaling that previously unfeasible studies are now possible. For example, the development of CRISPR gene editing, single-cell sequencing, and large language models each sparked waves of new research; AI can help researchers identify the next such catalysts earlier in their development cycle.

OPTIMIZING EXPERIMENTAL DESIGN

Once hypotheses are formulated, researchers face the challenge of designing studies to test them effectively and thoroughly. This is where AI's computational strengths are most useful: the design space for even moderately complex studies is large, and systematically exploring that space can uncover options that human intuition alone might overlook.

DESIGN SPACE EXPLORATION

A research design involves numerous decisions, causing combinations to increase rapidly. AI can generate various design options that address the same research question, allowing researchers to explicitly compare tradeoffs rather than settling on the first suitable design they find. This process can consider multiple constraints at once, such as budget, timeline, feasibility, statistical power, and ethical requirements, and identify designs that meet all of them, or determine exactly how much each constraint needs to be relaxed to create a feasible design.

Tradeoff analysis is especially useful. How much statistical power is gained by increasing the sample size from 200 to 300 compared to adding a second measurement time point? What is the participant burden cost of switching from a between-subject to a within-subject design, and does the power increase justify it? How sensitive are the conclusions about the design to assumptions about effect sizes or attrition rates? These questions can be addressed through systematic simulation before collecting any data, helping researchers allocate their resources where they will have the greatest impact.

FACTORIAL AND MEASUREMENT DESIGN

For experiments involving multiple factors, design complexity increases rapidly. Full factorial designs that combine all factor levels with each other quickly become impractical; fractional factorial approaches that test carefully selected combinations can recover most information at a lower cost, but determining which combinations to include is a combinatorial optimization problem well-suited to AI.[7] Response surface methodology, which maps how outcomes change across continuous factor levels to find optimal conditions, also benefits from algorithmic optimization of where to sample in the factor space.

Measurement design choices are equally important. Which variables are most crucial to measure, considering research goals and practical limitations? When should outcomes be evaluated, how often, and with what intervals? Should multiple measurement methods be combined to enhance construct validity? For biomedical studies, which biomarkers should be selected based on biological plausibility, practicality, and cost? AI can assist researchers in systematically evaluating these decisions by using data from similar studies to guide what to measure and when.

SAMPLE SIZE AND POWER CALCULATIONS

Deciding how many participants to recruit is one of the most important design choices, with direct effects on statistical power, feasibility, cost, and ethics. Underpowered studies waste resources by yielding inconclusive results; overpowered studies waste resources by recruiting more participants than needed, exposing people to research procedures without proportional scientific benefit.

Traditional power analysis requires researchers to define expected effect sizes, a task that is both essential and notoriously challenging. AI can enhance this process by analyzing existing literature to generate more precise effect size estimates than researcher intuition alone can offer, as well as by quantifying the uncertainty surrounding those estimates to demonstrate how power calculations vary across plausible ranges.[8] For complex designs with multiple outcomes, AI can compute power for each hypothesis concurrently and identify the minimum sample size necessary for all key tests.

When analytical power formulas are unavailable, especially for complex or nonstandard designs, simulation-based methods provide an alternative. Monte Carlo simulation creates synthetic datasets under different scenarios to empirically estimate power, and AI can automate this process across hundreds of scenarios. This helps test how assumption violations (such as nonnormality, heteroscedasticity, or different missing data patterns) impact power and compare the effectiveness of various analytical strategies to guide method choice.

Bayesian methods for determining sample size provide an alternative approach. Instead of aiming for a specific hypothesis-testing power level, researchers can base sample sizes on the precision of effect estimates they want or develop sequential designs that allow stopping data collection once enough evidence is gathered.[9] These methods are especially useful when prior knowledge exists and when the expense of gathering additional data is significant.

Throughout, decisions about sample size must be based on practical realities. AI can help combine budget constraints (what can we afford?), timeline limitations (how quickly can we recruit?), population availability (are enough eligible participants accessible?), and expected attrition (how many will complete the study?) into a single optimization that balances statistical goals with real-world feasibility.

ADAPTIVE TRIAL DESIGN

Traditional research designs are fixed before data collection begins: the sample size, randomization scheme, and analysis plan are specified in advance and followed regardless of growing results. Adaptive designs break this mold by allowing preplanned adjustments based on interim data while preserving statistical validity, and AI is increasingly vital in making these designs feasible.

CORE ADAPTIVE STRATEGIES

Response-adaptive randomization modifies the chance of assignment to different study arms as evidence builds, guiding more participants toward better-performing treatments.[10] This offers both statistical and ethical benefits: more participants receive effective treatments, and the trial learns more about promising options. Covariate-adaptive randomization keeps balance on key prognostic factors, while biomarker-adaptive assignment uses emerging biomarker-outcome links to steer enrollment toward participants most likely to benefit, a crucial component of precision medicine trials.

Sample size reestimation addresses a common problem in research design: the assumptions used for initial power calculations often turn out to be incorrect. Adaptive designs can update sample size estimates as real outcome variance becomes known, adjust targets if interim results indicate effects differ from initial assumptions, and apply stopping rules either for futility (if evidence suggests the intervention is unlikely to work) or for superiority (if evidence of benefit surpasses preset thresholds). These adjustments can save considerable time and resources while protecting participants from unnecessary exposure to ineffective interventions.

Population enrichment designs advance adaptation by adjusting enrollment criteria based on interim results. If early data indicate that an intervention is effective only in a specific subgroup, enrollment can be targeted to that group, increasing the likelihood of detecting effects where they truly occur. Seamless phase designs integrate traditionally separate research phases, such as dose-finding and efficacy testing or safety and preliminary efficacy assessments, into a single adaptive framework. This reduces gaps between phases and speeds up the research process.[11]

AI'S ESSENTIAL ROLE

Adaptive designs are conceptually elegant but logistically challenging. They require real-time analysis of accumulating data, quick decision-making on modifications, and careful statistical management to prevent adaptations from introducing bias. AI supports all of these tasks: analyzing interim data to guide adaptation decisions, simulating the operating characteristics of proposed adaptive designs before trial start (ensuring they maintain valid error rates across various scenarios), and optimizing stopping rules and modification triggers.

A 2025 perspective in npj Digital Medicine emphasized how AI is speeding up this integration, noting that reinforcement learning algorithms can now support real-time protocol adjustments, while digital twin modeling allows in silico testing of design changes before they are applied with real participants.[12] The combination of adaptive trial methods with AI-driven decision support is one of the most promising advances in clinical research, but it also increases the need for transparent reporting and regulatory oversight.

AI AS A CREATIVE RESEARCH PARTNER

Beyond optimizing predetermined design parameters, AI can act as a truly creative partner in methodological innovation, proposing approaches that researchers working within their field's conventions might not consider.

AI can suggest unconventional factor combinations in factorial designs, recommend alternative control strategies that strengthen causal inference, or create hybrid designs that combine elements of different types in new ways. For measurement, AI can suggest multimodal assessment methods that integrate self-report, behavioral observation, physiological monitoring, and digital traces to capture constructs more fully than any single approach. It can optimize the timing and frequency of ecological momentary assessments to balance the value of information with participant burden[13] and find opportunities to use passive data collection (smartphone sensors and digital traces) to measure constructs that usually require active, invasive assessment.

Perhaps most valuable, AI can identify methodological parallels across different fields. A research challenge in psychology may have been solved with an innovative design in ecology; a measurement method common in engineering might be unfamiliar in public health but still directly useful. By examining methodological descriptions across large bodies of literature, AI can reveal these cross-domain connections in ways no individual researcher, no matter how well-read, could match.

ANTICIPATING AND ADDRESSING METHODOLOGICAL CHALLENGES

Experienced researchers understand that the space between a study protocol and its implementation often leads to difficulties. AI can assist in predicting these issues beforehand, allowing for proactive solutions instead of reactive fixes.

Recruitment challenges lead to more study failures than any other factor. AI can estimate realistic enrollment rates based on target population traits and eligibility criteria from similar past studies, identify barriers that have hindered recruitment in comparable situations, and provide evidence-based timeline estimates. Missing data, the second most common threat to study validity, can be proactively managed through AI-driven prediction of likely missingness patterns, identification of successful prevention strategies from similar contexts, and planning appropriate analytical methods for the inevitable missing data.

AI can also assist with anticipating protocol deviations, measurement issues (such as ceiling and floor effects, response burden, and order effects), and challenges in coordinating across multiple sites by reviewing what went well and what did not in similar past studies. For multisite studies, AI can improve site selection by evaluating recruitment capacity, geographic diversity, technical infrastructure, and complementary strengths among potential sites. Additionally, AI can help plan the data harmonization procedures needed when integrating measurements collected differently across locations.

ETHICAL CONSIDERATIONS IN RESEARCH DESIGN

Research design decisions have significant ethical implications, and AI can assist researchers in addressing these considerations more systematically, though it cannot determine the underlying value judgments.

Minimizing participant burden is both an ethical responsibility and a practical necessity for recruitment and retention. AI can measure the total burden from all study procedures and identify ways to improve efficiency, helping to achieve research goals with less participant time and effort. For clinical trials, assessing equipoise, ensuring that the proposed comparisons truly reflect scientific uncertainty, can be guided by AI synthesis of existing evidence. However, determining whether genuine equipoise exists still requires clinical expertise that AI cannot provide.

Justice in study design requires that research be conducted fairly. AI can identify when proposed eligibility criteria might systematically exclude disadvantaged groups, when study procedures may not be culturally appropriate for target populations, or when the populations bearing research burdens differ from those likely to benefit from the results. Privacy considerations, data minimization, deidentification planning, and disclosure risk assessment can be handled more systematically with AI support, especially as studies increasingly gather sensitive digital data.

An emerging concern related to AI-supported design is the risk of algorithmic bias. If AI learns optimal designs from historical patterns, it may replicate biases present in past research: measurement methods that work well for majority populations but poorly for minorities, recruitment strategies that miss hard-to-reach groups, and analytical choices that favor statistical convenience over scientific thoroughness. Researchers need to critically assess AI design suggestions for these hidden biases rather than accepting them as neutral improvements.

PRACTICAL IMPLEMENTATION STRATEGIES

Effective use of AI for hypothesis generation and research design depends on starting with domain knowledge and using AI to augment, not replace, expert judgment. Theory-informed hypothesis generation employs AI to identify patterns within frameworks suggested by existing theory, rather than engaging in random data exploration. Methodological expertise guarantees that AI-designed approaches are practical in real-world settings. Iterative refinement, including generating multiple design options, gathering stakeholder feedback, and conducting pilot tests of key assumptions, produces more robust designs than simply accepting AI's initial recommendation.

Transparency remains crucial throughout the process. When AI influences design decisions, researchers should clearly state its role, explain why specific features were selected, document what alternatives were considered, and describe the assumptions behind AI analyses. This openness enhances both reproducibility and trust, allowing other researchers to assess and expand on AI-informed design choices.

Verification is also important. AI-generated power calculations should be verified with independent analysis. Adaptive designs informed by AI simulation need validation through separate simulation runs. Methodological experts should review AI-informed designs before they are implemented. These verification steps are not just formalities; they are safeguards against overconfidence that can stem from AI's ability to produce sophisticated-looking outputs, regardless of their actual quality.

CAPABILITIES AND LIMITATIONS: THE DESIGN AND HYPOTHESIS AUDIT

While the Master Matrix in Chapter 1 outlines general AI strengths in Pattern Recognition and Code and Scripting, applying these to hypothesis generation and study design requires specific Override Triggers. In this phase, the transition from "correlation" to "causation" is where AI models are most likely to fail. Designing a study is a clinical art that requires human wisdom to balance competing values, a task far beyond algorithmic optimization (Table 5.1).

TABLE 5.1
Design-Specific Override Protocols

Design Task	AI Execution (The "Meat")	The Human Override (The Top Bread)
Pattern discovery	Spotting nonobvious correlations across massive multiomic or clinical datasets	**Mechanistic Validation:** Humans must determine *why* a relationship exists. AI cannot distinguish between a biological breakthrough and a spurious correlation
Power analysis	Rapidly calculating sample size requirements across dozens of hypothetical scenarios	**Clinical Significance Audit:** Humans must define the "Effect Size." AI can calculate statistical power, but it cannot judge what constitutes a *meaningful* difference in a patient's life
Bias screening	Systematically checking protocols against known bias frameworks (e.g., selection or attrition bias)	**Contextual Adaptation:** AI identifies "textbook" biases; humans must identify "local" biases specific to their patient population or clinical site

(*Continued*)

TABLE 5.1 (*Continued*)
Design-Specific Override Protocols

Design Task	AI Execution (The "Meat")	The Human Override (The Top Bread)
Outcome simulation	Modeling study results under various assumptions to optimize trial arms	**Plausibility Check:** Review AI-simulated "successes" against known physiological laws. If the simulation violates biological reality, the model parameters must be manually reset

Refer to the Master Matrix in Chapter 1 for foundational failure modes; the table outlines the expert-level interventions required for study design.

The "Correlational Cul-de-Sac"

A primary limitation in AI-assisted hypothesis generation is its inability to perform Causal Reasoning. AI identifies variables that move together, but it lacks the theoretical understanding to explain the underlying mechanism.

- **The AI Limit**: AI may suggest a hypothesis based on a strong statistical link that is actually a "confounding by indication" or a quirk of the training data.
- **The Human Task**: You must provide the "Theoretical Anchor." Use AI to surface patterns but trigger a Manual Override to ensure every proposed hypothesis aligns with established (or plausibly emerging) biological mechanisms.

DESIGN TRADEOFFS AND "GROUNDING IN THE DIRT"

Study design is a series of compromises between internal validity (rigor) and external validity (real-world applicability). AI can optimize for *numbers*, but it cannot optimize for *values*.

1. **Ethics versus Power**: AI may suggest a larger sample size to achieve statistical "perfection" without accounting for the ethical burden on a rare-disease population or the limited pool of eligible participants.
2. **The Art of Feasibility**: AI-generated designs are often "clinically sterile." They fail to account for the "messiness" of human research, such as the likelihood of patient drop-off during holiday seasons or the technical difficulty of a specific imaging sequence.
3. **The "Wrong Question" Risk**: No amount of AI optimization can salvage a study designed to answer a question that doesn't matter to the clinical community or the funding agency.

The Override Trigger: If the AI suggests a "perfect" study design that requires resources, timelines, or participant compliance levels that exceed your local institutional reality, you must trigger a Feasibility Bypass. You are the final judge of what is "doable"; the AI is merely a simulator of what is "possible."

THE SKEPTIC'S CORNER

- **Target Task**: Experimental design and power analysis.
- **Adversarial Prompt**: "Identify three 'black box' assumptions in the experimental design you just suggested. Which specific confounding variables are likely to invalidate this model if the data is collected in a real-world clinical setting rather than a controlled lab?"

LOOKING FORWARD

AI capabilities for supporting research design continue to progress on multiple fronts. Integrated design platforms that combine hypothesis generation, design optimization, power analysis, and simulation within unified workflows are emerging, reducing the difficulty of switching between separate tools for each decision.

Real-time adaptive learning systems that continuously optimize based on accumulating data, rather than following fixed adaptation rules, promise more flexible and efficient trial execution. Multiobjective optimization is becoming more advanced, managing competing design goals such as power, cost, burden, and generalizability with greater nuance. The integration of causal inference frameworks into AI-supported design is enhancing researchers' ability to move beyond mere associations toward truly causal hypotheses.

The International Conference on Learning Representations 2025 workshop on "Agentic AI for Science" emphasized a broader goal: fully autonomous AI systems capable of generating hypotheses, designing experiments, and validating results with minimal human input.[14] Although this vision still seems distant and its desirability is debated, the near-term trend is clear: AI will increasingly act as a capable research partner that handles computational and pattern-recognition tasks, allowing human researchers to focus on the creative, strategic, and ethical aspects of study design that remain their unique contribution.

CONCLUSION

The shift from research questions to rigorous study designs demands creativity, technical skill, and careful judgment of competing values. AI provides powerful tools to support each part of this process: spotting patterns that suggest hypotheses, systematically exploring complex design options, optimizing sample sizes and adaptive features, and helping to foresee implementation challenges.

These capabilities work best when paired with domain expertise, theoretical knowledge, and human judgment about which questions matter and what tradeoffs are acceptable. AI broadens the design space researchers can explore and helps them make more informed methodological choices, but it cannot replace the creative and ethical reasoning vital to good research design. The researchers who gain the most will be those who view AI as a capable collaborator, one whose contributions demand the same careful evaluation as any other source of input.

The next chapter examines how AI can assist with research program and portfolio optimization, helping institutions and funders make strategic decisions regarding research investments across various studies and investigators.

KEY TAKEAWAYS

- AI pattern recognition in existing data can generate hypotheses by identifying unexpected associations, subgroup effects, and temporal patterns, but these require prospective testing and theoretical grounding.
- The largest empirical test to date found that AI-generated hypotheses are meaningful and testable but still lag behind human ones in novelty and experimental success.
- AI-driven design optimization allows systematic exploration of complex design spaces, quantifying tradeoffs that researchers would otherwise rely on intuition to navigate.
- Sample size determination benefits from AI-powered literature mining for effect sizes, simulation-based power analysis for complex designs, and the integration of practical constraints.
- Adaptive trial designs, including response-adaptive randomization, sample size reestimation, and population enrichment, become more practical with AI support for real-time decision-making.
- Cross-domain methodological transfer, enabled by AI analysis of methods across fields, is an underutilized source of design innovation.
- Ethical design involves balancing statistical efficiency with participant welfare, fairness, and scientific values, tradeoffs that AI can help clarify but humans must ultimately decide.
- Transparency regarding AI's role in design development is crucial for reproducibility and trust.

QUESTIONS FOR REFLECTION

1. What patterns in existing data relevant to your research might be worth investigating as testable hypotheses, and how would you differentiate real signals from statistical artifacts?
2. How can AI-supported design optimization assist you in balancing competing priorities like power, feasibility, cost, and participant burden in your research?
3. What design innovations from other fields could be effectively adapted to questions in your area?
4. How would you make sure that AI-supported design stays grounded in theory and feasibility constraints?
5. What ethical considerations are most important in your research context, and how might AI assist or impede in addressing them?
6. If AI can create and improve study designs, what is the researcher's unique contribution, and how should authorship of the design be assigned?

NOTES

1. Pushpakom, S., Iorio F., Eyers, P. A., Escott, K. J., Hopper, S., Wells, A., Doig, A., Guilliams, T., Latimer, J., McNamee, C., Norris, A., Sanseau, P., Cavalla, D., & Pirmohamed, M. (2019). Drug repurposing: Progress, challenges and recommendations. *Nature Reviews Drug Discovery,* 18(1), 41–58. https://doi.org/10.1038/nrd.2018.168. Epub 2018 Oct 12. PMID: 30310233. Note: This review covers AI-driven and computational approaches to drug repurposing using electronic health records, insurance claims data, and multiomics integration, providing extensive examples of hypothesis generation from secondary data analysis.
2. Hasin, Y., Seldin, M., & Lusis, A. (2017). Multi-omics approaches to disease. *Genome Biology*, 18(1), 83. https://doi.org/10.1186/s13059-017-1215-1
3. van der Maaten, L., & Hinton, G. (2008). Visualizing data using t-SNE. *Journal of Machine Learning Research*, 9, 2579–2605. http://www.jmlr.org/papers/v9/vandermaaten08a.html
4. Sun, D., et al. (2025). AI-assisted hypothesis generation to address challenges in cardiotoxicity research. *Journal of Medical Internet Research*, 27, e66161. https://doi.org/10.2196/66161

5. Gottweis, J., et al. (2025). Towards an AI co-scientist. arXiv:2502.18864. https://arxiv.org/abs/2502.18864. See also: Google Research. (2025, February 18). Accelerating scientific breakthroughs with an AI co-scientist. https://research.google/blog/accelerating-scientific-breakthroughs-with-an-ai-co-scientist/
6. Brainard, J. (2025, August 24). AI-generated scientific hypotheses lag human ones when put to the test. *Science*. https://www.science.org/content/article/ai-generated-scientific-hypotheses-lag-human-ones-when-put-test. Note: *Science* news article reporting on the article by Si, C. et al. (2024/2025). Can LLMs Generate Novel Research Ideas? A Large-Scale Human Study with 100+ NLP Researchers. *arXiv preprint*. https://arxiv.org/abs/2409.04109.
7. Montgomery, D. C. (2017). *Design and Analysis of Experiments* (9th ed.). Wiley.
8. Lakens, D. (2022). Sample size justification. *Collabra: Psychology*, 8(1), 33267. https://doi.org/10.1525/collabra.33267
9. Spiegelhalter, D. J., Abrams, K. R., & Myles, J. P. (2004). *Bayesian Approaches to Clinical Trials and Health-Care Evaluation*. Wiley.
10. Thall, P. F., & Wathen, J. K. (2007). Practical Bayesian adaptive randomisation in clinical trials. *European Journal of Cancer*, 43(5), 859–866. https://doi.org/10.1016/j.ejca.2007.01.006
11. Woodcock, J., & LaVange, L. M. (2017). Master protocols to study multiple therapies, multiple diseases, or both. *New England Journal of Medicine*, 377(1), 62–70. https://doi.org/10.1056/NEJMra1510062
12. Sezgin, E., et al. (2025). AI and innovation in clinical trials. *NPJ Digital Medicine*, 8(1), 683. https://doi.org/10.1038/s41746-025-02048-5. Note: This perspective examines AI-driven eligibility optimization, reinforcement learning for real-time adaptation, and digital twin modeling for in silico trial testing.
13. Shiffman, S., Stone, A. A., & Hufford, M. R. (2008). Ecological momentary assessment. *Annual Review of Clinical Psychology*, 4, 1–32. https://doi.org/10.1146/annurev.clinpsy.3.022806.091415
14. ICLR 2025 Workshop: Towards agentic AI for science: Hypothesis generation, experiment design, and scientific discovery. https://iclr.cc/virtual/2025/workshop/23991. Note: This multi-speaker workshop explored integrating agentic AI systems into scientific discovery while maintaining rigorous standards for hypothesis validation and experimental feasibility. The conference abstract was submitted by: Danai Koutra, Lifu Huang, Adithya Kulkarni, Temiloluwa Prioleau, Beatrice Soh, Qingyun Wu, Yujun Yan, Yaoqing Yang, Dawei Zhou, James Y Zou.

Part III

Research Management and Administration

6 AI for Biomedical Research Program and Portfolio Optimization

THE CHALLENGE OF RESEARCH PORTFOLIO MANAGEMENT

Research organizations, whether academic institutions, government agencies, foundations, or industry R&D departments, manage portfolios of multiple research programs, projects, and investigators. The challenge of managing these portfolios effectively is significant, and the stakes are high: decisions about how to allocate limited resources across competing research priorities influence what knowledge is generated, which diseases are studied, which communities benefit from research, and ultimately how much collective value the research enterprise produces.

Effective portfolio management involves balancing considerations that often pull in opposite directions. Strategic alignment requires that research portfolios support organizational missions and stakeholder needs, yet the most transformative discoveries often come from work that no strategic plan predicted. Resource allocation must distribute funding, facilities, and personnel across competing priorities, but the information needed to make optimal choices, such as which projects will succeed, which will have impact, and which synergies will develop, is inherently uncertain at the time decisions are made. Risk management involves balancing high-risk, high-reward research that could transform fields with steadier work that

DOI 10.1201/9781003782995-9

produces consistent progress and maintains organizational stability, though these categories are not always clearly distinguishable in advance. Additionally, diversification must maintain breadth across topics, methods, career stages, and populations studied, without dispersing resources so thinly that nothing reaches critical mass.

These challenges have become more severe in recent years. The National Institutes of Health funding environment described in Chapter 3, with R01-equivalent success rates dropping to about 20% and the lump-sum funding policy limiting new awards, means that institutional portfolio choices have greater impacts than before. A poorly aligned portfolio can leave an institution without the competitive edge needed to secure funding in an increasingly competitive environment. Meanwhile, the amount of data available about research activities has grown tremendously: publication databases, citation networks, grant databases, patent filings, clinical trial registries, and Altmetric platforms collectively hold extensive information about what research is being done, by whom, where, and with what outcomes.

Traditional portfolio management depends heavily on leadership experience, expert judgment, periodic strategic planning exercises, and qualitative evaluation of research quality and impact. These remain crucial, as no algorithm can replace a dean's understanding of institutional culture or a program officer's judgment of which investigators can produce transformative work. However, artificial intelligence (AI) can offer complementary analytical support that makes portfolio decisions more systematic, transparent, and evidence-based. This chapter examines where that support is most beneficial.

STRATEGIC RESEARCH PLANNING

Strategic planning for research portfolios starts with understanding the environment in which the organization operates, including what other institutions are doing, where funding is flowing, what technologies are emerging, and how societal needs are evolving.

ENVIRONMENTAL SCANNING AND OPPORTUNITY IDENTIFICATION

AI-powered environmental scanning far surpasses what any individual or small team can do manually. The emerging field of "science of science," which employs computational methods to analyze how scientific research evolves, provides the intellectual basis for many of these capabilities.[1] By examining publication trends, citation patterns, funding flows, and collaboration networks at scale, AI can identify which research areas are expanding, maturing, or declining globally; uncover what peer institutions are investing in and where opportunities for differentiation exist; monitor changing priorities among major funding agencies; and spot emerging technologies that will open new research avenues.

These analyses become strategically valuable when they move beyond mere description to provide actionable insights. For example, AI might identify that a competitor institution has recently hired three faculty members in a specific area, signaling a strategic commitment, information that helps decide whether to compete directly, seek collaboration, or differentiate into an adjacent niche. Alternatively, analysis might show that a particular research area is producing more publications but fewer citations per paper, indicating a maturing field where entering might be less attractive than publication volume alone suggests.

Opportunity identification extends further. AI can detect emerging research areas before they become mainstream by recognizing accelerating cocitation patterns or shifts in terminology. It can also identify where different research strengths within an organization might be productively combined in ways that haven't been explored yet and uncover latent capabilities, areas where an institution has relevant expertise that could be activated with targeted investment. For translational research, AI can map where organizational capabilities align with unmet clinical needs or commercial opportunities, linking basic science strengths to potential applications.

STRATEGIC POSITIONING ANALYSIS

Understanding where an organization stands relative to competitors and collaborators informs every strategic decision. AI can assess competitive advantages by analyzing publication impact, funding success rates, and collaboration centrality across research domains, identifying areas where the institution genuinely leads versus areas where it merely participates. Differentiation opportunities emerge when AI reveals niches that no competitor currently occupies but that align with organizational strengths. And the necessity of collaboration becomes apparent when analysis shows that meaningful contributions to certain research areas require partnerships rather than independent work, a finding that can redirect resources from futile competition toward productive alliance-building.

PORTFOLIO ANALYSIS AND DIVERSIFICATION

Understanding what a research portfolio currently includes and excludes is essential for its improvement. AI provides this understanding with a level of detail and systematic analysis that manual assessment cannot match.

COMPOSITION AND CONCENTRATION ANALYSIS

AI can analyze a research portfolio across multiple dimensions at once: thematic distribution (how resources are spread across topics and questions), methodological diversity (the variety of research approaches used), population coverage (which groups are studied and which are overlooked), career stage distribution (the mix of established and early-career investigators), collaboration patterns (internal and external networks), and funding source diversity (dependence on certain revenue streams versus broader diversification).

This multidimensional mapping often uncovers surprising patterns. An institution might find that despite a stated commitment to health disparities research, less than 5% of its portfolio focuses on underserved populations. Or, analysis might show that while the institution employs researchers using diverse methods, collaboration between different methodological traditions is rare, a missed opportunity for mixed-methods innovation. These insights are hard to produce through qualitative assessment alone because they require synthesizing information across hundreds of projects and investigators.

Concentration risk is a particular concern. When too many resources are invested in narrow areas, the portfolio becomes vulnerable to shifts in the field, funding changes, or the departure of key investigators.[2] AI can quantify concentration across all portfolio dimensions and highlight areas where risk exceeds prudent thresholds. The analogy to financial portfolio diversification is imperfect; research is not a financial asset class, and "risk" in research has dimensions that financial models don't capture, but the main idea that diversification reduces vulnerability still applies. Understanding which research areas tend to succeed or struggle together (similar to asset correlation) helps inform diversification strategies: investing in research areas whose fortunes are independent offers better risk reduction than spreading resources across areas that tend to rise and fall together.

RESOURCE ALLOCATION AND PRIORITIZATION

Limited resources require tough allocation decisions, and these choices are among the most important that research leaders face. AI can make these decisions more systematic and transparent, though it cannot, and should not, make them automatically.

ALLOCATION FRAMEWORKS AND MODELING

Different philosophical frameworks influence resource allocation, and organizations must decide which to prioritize: maximizing expected impact, aligning with strategic goals, investing where they have competitive advantages, responding to emerging opportunities, ensuring fair distribution, or addressing overlooked needs. In reality, organizations often use multiple frameworks at once, and the tension among them creates difficult decisions. AI's role is to help organizations apply these frameworks consistently and make the tradeoffs explicit rather than implicit.

Resource allocation modeling converts strategic goals into specific scenarios. Based on stated objectives and constraints, optimization algorithms can identify allocations that maximize desired outcomes, compare how different strategies impact portfolio characteristics, evaluate the additional benefit of investing more resources in certain areas versus others, and find allocations that meet multiple requirements such as strategic priorities, diversity goals, infrastructure use, and budget limits. Multicriteria decision analysis offers a structured way to assess research areas across various aspects (scientific merit, feasibility, impact potential, and strategic fit) and identify the highest-priority investments.[3]

The value of these models lies not in their outputs being "correct," the inputs are too uncertain for that, but in making assumptions explicit, forcing systematic consideration of alternatives, and providing a common framework for stakeholders with different perspectives to engage in productive debate about priorities.

PREDICTING RESEARCH IMPACT AND RETURN ON INVESTMENT

Understanding likely research outcomes helps inform strategic decisions, but prediction in research is inherently uncertain, and the most important outcomes are often the least predictable.

WHAT CAN BE ESTIMATED

AI has demonstrated real ability in certain prediction tasks. Citation impact estimation, for example, relies on significant empirical work showing that publication impact can be partly predicted from the research's features, the investigators, and the publication venue.[4] Funding leverage prediction, which estimates how initial investments lead to subsequent external support, can utilize institutional track records and similar programs. Translation probability estimation can identify features of research programs that have historically resulted in clinical applications, patents, or policy influence, although with broad confidence intervals.

WHAT CANNOT BE PREDICTED

Several fundamental limits restrict research outcome prediction, and portfolio managers who overlook these limits risk making poorer decisions than they would with simpler methods. Breakthrough discoveries are inherently unpredictable; if we could forecast them, they wouldn't be true breakthroughs. The impact of research often shows up over years or decades, making short-term predictions unreliable. Predictions based on past patterns might not reflect changing technologies, funding environments, or societal needs. Easily measurable outcomes, like publications and citations, may not accurately represent the most important results, such as lives saved, policy changes, or social benefits. Perhaps most dangerously, if predictions influence how resources are allocated, they could create self-fulfilling prophecies: research areas predicted to succeed receive more support and therefore do succeed, regardless of their true potential, while those predicted to underperform are deprived of resources and tend to underperform.

For these reasons, impact predictions should guide rather than dictate portfolio decisions, with significant emphasis on expert judgment, strategic values, and intentional investment in unpredictable but potentially transformative work.

BALANCING RISK AND INNOVATION

Research portfolios must balance stability with innovation, steady and reliable progress with the potential for transformative breakthroughs. This balance is one of the most important and challenging aspects of portfolio management, and it is an area where AI can offer analytical structure to what is often an entirely intuitive process.

RISK-RETURN ANALYSIS

Portfolio theory from finance provides a useful, if imperfect, conceptual framework. The efficient frontier concept identifies portfolio combinations that maximize expected impact for a given level of risk: portfolios below the frontier are suboptimal because they accept more risk than necessary for their expected return or generate less return than possible for their risk level.[5] Research on how novelty and convention interact in scientific impact suggests that the most impactful work often combines conventional approaches with atypical elements, a finding that has direct implications for portfolio construction.[6]

Applying this framework to research requires recognizing its limitations. Research "risk" is multidimensional (technical, feasibility, impact uncertainty, opportunity cost, and reputational) in ways that financial risk is not. "Return" in research includes scientific knowledge, clinical applications, policy influence, economic benefits, and social outcomes that cannot be summarized by a single metric. Additionally, the time horizons of research impact are much longer and more unpredictable than financial returns. Despite these challenges, the framework offers valuable discipline: it compels portfolio managers to consider explicitly what risk level they accept, whether they are being compensated with potential impact for that risk, and if diversification across research programs truly reduces risk.

INNOVATION VERSUS INCREMENTAL RESEARCH

Both transformative innovation and steady incremental progress are vital to a healthy research portfolio, and the balance between them should be a deliberate strategic choice rather than a coincidence. AI can assist by evaluating how much of a portfolio genuinely challenges current paradigms versus how much it builds on established approaches, measuring the combined impact of incremental work (which is often underestimated in strategic discussions that focus on "moonshot" research), and simulating how different ratios of innovation to incremental work influence long-term portfolio results under various scenarios.

Strategic risk-taking, or making calculated bets on research with high uncertainty but strong rationale, is easier to justify when the overall portfolio offers stability. This is the key insight of portfolio diversification applied to research: an institution can afford to take bold risks on individual projects when the entire portfolio is resilient enough to handle failures.

GAP ANALYSIS AND CAPABILITY MAPPING

Understanding what an institution does well and what it doesn't do at all is essential for strategic positioning. AI provides this understanding at a level of detail that manual assessment rarely reaches.

RESEARCH GAP IDENTIFICATION

Gaps in research portfolios take many forms. Population gaps happen when certain communities are consistently understudied despite institutional mission commitments. Methodological gaps occur when potentially valuable research approaches are underused. Topic gaps arise when questions central to the organization's mission are not actively explored. Geographic gaps appear in global health or international research portfolios. Career stage gaps reflect imbalances in support for investigators at different stages of their careers. AI can identify each of these gaps by comparing portfolio contents against mission statements, peer institution portfolios, disease burden data, or stakeholder-identified priorities.

CAPABILITY MAPPING AND STRATEGIC ASSESSMENT

Mapping organizational capabilities uncovers not only current strengths but also potential that could be unlocked with targeted investment. Core competencies, areas of deep, distinctive expertise, can be identified through bibliometric analysis, funding success patterns, and collaboration centrality.[7,8] However, some of the most valuable strategic insights come from discovering hidden strengths: latent capabilities relevant to new research areas, cross-cutting competencies spanning multiple departments, or areas where modest additional investment could transform marginal capabilities into distinctive advantages.

Honest identification of weaknesses is equally crucial. Recognizing capability gaps, resource limitations, and strategic mismatches helps organizations avoid overextending themselves and directs investments to where they can truly excel. The desire to expand into every promising area is strong; AI-informed capability mapping provides the discipline to resist this urge.

MULTIOBJECTIVE OPTIMIZATION

Research portfolio decisions involve multiple, often competing objectives, such as scientific discovery, clinical translation, workforce development, equity, and sustainability, and no single optimization can satisfy all of them simultaneously.

NAVIGATING TRADEOFFS

The main contribution of multiobjective optimization is making tradeoffs clear. Short-term productivity might clash with building long-term capabilities. Covering many areas might conflict with developing deep expertise. Taking risks could threaten organizational stability. Supporting star investigators might conflict with providing opportunities broadly. Each of these tensions is real, and pretending they don't exist, or solving them secretly through bureaucratic inertia, leads to worse results than facing them directly.

Pareto analysis offers a solid framework for this comparison. By pinpointing the efficient frontier, which is the set of portfolio compositions where improving one goal means sacrificing another, Pareto analysis removes clearly inferior options and directs decision-makers' focus to real tradeoffs. AI can calculate these frontiers across many dimensions at once, showing the rate at which objectives must be balanced against each other and aiding decision-makers in understanding the outcomes of different choices.

Ultimately, however, choosing among points on the efficient frontier is a matter of values, not analysis. AI can clarify the tradeoffs involved; humans must decide which ones to accept. Preference elicitation techniques, structured processes for determining how much different objectives matter, what constraints are absolute, and which scenarios are preferred, can assist organizations in revealing and aligning the implicit values that often influence portfolio decisions without being recognized.

COLLABORATIVE PORTFOLIO DEVELOPMENT

Research portfolios increasingly span institutions, disciplines, and sectors. Multiinstitutional research networks, consortium grants, and collaborative platforms create portfolios that no single organization controls, raising coordination challenges that AI can help solve.

AI can evaluate how different institutions' strengths complement each other, identify duplicative investments that indicate coordination opportunities, uncover coverage gaps that no single partner addresses, and assess whether contributions and benefits are fairly distributed among partners. Network analysis can identify investigators or institutions that act as bridges between otherwise disconnected research communities, as well as strategic structural positions worth supporting.[8] Information flow analysis can determine whether research findings circulate effectively across networks or become trapped in isolated clusters, highlighting where intentional knowledge-sharing mechanisms are needed.

IMPLEMENTATION AND CHANGE MANAGEMENT

Portfolio optimization suggestions are only as useful as their execution, and making strategic changes to research portfolios is inherently challenging. Research portfolios have significant inertia: investigators have dedicated careers to specific research areas, infrastructure has been established for particular goals, and funding commitments extend years ahead.

A phased implementation is crucial. AI can assist in sequencing changes by pinpointing which portfolio adjustments yield the greatest strategic benefit with minimal disruption, planning resource shifts that honor existing commitments while gradually moving toward new priorities, and identifying quick wins that garner organizational support for larger changes. Continuous stakeholder engagement is essential: researchers affected by reduced emphasis need transparent communication, involvement in planning processes, and support during transitions. Imposing portfolio strategies without consultation fosters resistance and distrust, undermining even well-designed plans.

Continuous monitoring closes the gap between strategy and execution. AI can track whether portfolio development aligns with goals, assess whether strategic investments deliver expected outcomes, identify environmental shifts that require strategic adjustments, and support the adaptive management essential to any long-term strategy.

ETHICAL CONSIDERATIONS

Portfolio optimization raises deep ethical questions that technical analysis cannot solve. Equity requires that research portfolios serve diverse populations rather than only those that are easiest to study or most commercially attractive, provide fair opportunities across researcher demographics and career stages, and avoid the systematic neglect of questions important to marginalized communities. These are not just constraints to be satisfied and forgotten; they are values that should influence every portfolio decision.

Scientific freedom creates a real tension with strategic direction. Investigator autonomy, the freedom to pursue intellectually compelling questions regardless of strategic fit, has historically led to many of science's most important discoveries. However, unrestricted autonomy can result in portfolios that overlook key societal needs, duplicate efforts, or fail to develop critical mass in any area. The solution is not to choose one value over the other but to maintain a deliberate balance: strategic direction for part of the portfolio, protected space for curiosity-driven exploration in another, and ongoing dialogue about where the boundary should be.

Perhaps most subtly, portfolio optimization can systematically bias toward what is measurable rather than what is truly important. Metrics-driven approaches favor research that yields immediate publications over slower-developing work with greater long-term impact, established areas with proven success over emerging fields with uncertain potential, and quantifiable outcomes over diffuse but meaningful societal contributions. Portfolio managers must explicitly value long-term, risky, and hard-to-measure research, or optimization will gradually push these efforts out.

CAPABILITIES AND LIMITATIONS: THE PORTFOLIO AUDIT

While the Master Matrix in Chapter 1 outlines general AI strengths in Pattern Analysis and Decision Support, applying these to research portfolio management requires a specialized set of Override Triggers. Portfolio optimization is not a purely mathematical exercise; it is a strategic and political one. AI can calculate the "balance" of a portfolio, but it cannot navigate the institutional culture or the long-term vision required to sustain it (Table 6.1).

TABLE 6.1
Portfolio-Specific Override Protocols

Portfolio Task	AI Execution (The "Meat")	The Human Override (The Top Bread)
Multiobjective optimization	Finding the "mathematical best" allocation across competing research goals	**Strategic Realignment:** Humans must decide which "goal" takes precedence when values conflict. AI cannot prioritize a mission over a metric
Scenario modeling	Forecasting how different investment strategies might perform under future market/funding conditions	**Plausibility Audit:** Review AI forecasts against current geopolitical and federal funding shifts (e.g., 2026 budget cycles). AI often relies on stale historical trends

(*Continued*)

TABLE 6.1 (*Continued*)
Portfolio-Specific Override Protocols

Portfolio Task	AI Execution (The "Meat")	The Human Override (The Top Bread)
Gap and overlap analysis	Comparing internal portfolios against benchmarks, missions, and peer institutions	**Niche Identification:** AI identifies *statistical* gaps; humans must identify *reputational* gaps. Decide if a gap represents an opportunity or a strategic distraction
Resource allocation	Suggesting distribution of funds, space, or personnel based on productivity metrics	**Culture Check:** Audit AI suggestions for "invisible" constraints, such as faculty morale, historical commitments, or specific lab synergies

Refer to the Master Matrix in Chapter 1 for foundational failure modes; the table outlines the expert-level interventions required for institutional leadership.

THE METRIC-FIXATION TRAP

A critical limitation in AI-driven portfolio management is the Quantification Bias. AI models excel at optimizing what can be measured (h-index, grant dollars, and publication counts) but are blind to what cannot be easily quantified, such as research excellence, mentorship quality, or institutional "goodwill."

- **The AI Limit**: AI can distinguish between "productive" and "unproductive" work, but it struggles to distinguish between "merely competent" work and "truly exceptional" work that has yet to yield metrics.
- **The Human Task**: You must provide the Qualitative Appraisal. Use AI to surface the data but trigger a Manual Override to protect high-potential, long-term research that may not yet satisfy a "short-term" algorithm.

POLITICAL NAVIGATION AND VISIONARY LEADERSHIP

Portfolio management is inherently a human-centric leadership task. AI lacks the "Institutional Intelligence" to:

1. **Navigate Politics**: AI cannot sense the interpersonal dynamics, historical grievances, or departmental rivalries that make a theoretically "optimal" plan practically impossible.
2. **Articulate Vision**: AI can show you what currently exists; it cannot inspire a team to build what *should* exist. Visionary leadership requires imagination and a "moral compass" that AI lacks.
3. **Manage Organizational Culture**: What succeeds at a large state university might fail at a private research institute. AI cannot "see" the cultural nuances that determine whether a strategic pivot will be embraced or resisted by the faculty.

The Override Trigger: If the AI suggests a "mathematically optimal" portfolio reorganization that ignores human relationships or institutional history, you must trigger a **Political Feasibility Bypass**. You are the final arbiter of strategic direction; the AI is merely an analyst of existing patterns.

THE SKEPTIC'S CORNER

- **Target Task:** Resource allocation and risk assessment.
- **Adversarial Prompt:** "This portfolio allocation maximizes 'expected impact' based on publication metrics. Now, argue that this allocation creates a 'self-fulfilling prophecy' that suppresses high-risk innovation, and show me how a budget shift would look if we prioritized 'scientific resilience' over 'citation volume'."

LOOKING FORWARD

AI capabilities for portfolio optimization continue to advance across multiple areas. Integrated platforms that combine portfolio analysis, resource allocation modeling, outcome tracking, and adaptive management into unified systems are emerging, reducing the fragmentation that currently limits institutional research intelligence. Real-time monitoring will enable more dynamic portfolio management, replacing annual strategic planning cycles with ongoing adjustments. Predictive abilities will get better, although fundamental uncertainty about research outcomes will always limit their usefulness. Network analysis will become more advanced, better capturing the collaborative dynamics that increasingly influence research productivity. Additionally, multi-stakeholder optimization methods will improve, helping institutions balance the perspectives of investigators, administrators, community partners, funders, and the public.

However, the fundamental nature of research portfolio management, making value-laden strategic decisions about collective research direction, will remain primarily human-led work. The institutions that succeed will be those that use AI to make their portfolio decisions more informed, transparent, and systematic while maintaining the human judgment, creativity, and ethical reasoning that no algorithm can replace.

CONCLUSION

Research portfolio management involves balancing many competing considerations: strategic priorities and emerging opportunities, risk and stability, efficiency and fairness, and short-term productivity and long-term impact. AI provides powerful analytical tools for these decisions: assessing current portfolios, identifying gaps and opportunities, modeling resource allocation scenarios, estimating research outcomes, and evaluating tradeoffs among competing objectives.

These capabilities can assist research organizations in making more informed strategic decisions, but they work best when combined with leadership vision, stakeholder input, and human judgment about values and priorities. AI can make portfolio management more transparent, analytical, and systematic, but it cannot replace the creative and ethical reasoning essential to strategic research leadership. The most effective approach treats AI as a tool for illuminating choices, not replacing them.

The next chapter discusses how AI can assist in team building and collaboration, helping researchers find and form successful partnerships for complex research projects.

KEY TAKEAWAYS

- Research portfolio management involves balancing strategic priorities, resource constraints, risk tolerance, and diverse stakeholder interests, with decisions carrying heightened consequences in the current tight funding environment.
- AI facilitates systematic portfolio analysis across multiple dimensions simultaneously, uncovering strengths, gaps, and concentration risks that are not evident from qualitative assessment alone.
- Resource allocation modeling clarifies tradeoffs between competing investment options, enabling more transparent and evidence-based decision-making.
- Research outcome prediction can inform but should never dictate portfolio decisions, considering fundamental uncertainties about breakthroughs and long-term impact.
- Risk-return analysis adapted from financial portfolio theory offers a useful discipline, although research "risk" and "return" are far more complex than their financial counterparts.
- Multiobjective Pareto optimization shows what tradeoffs are possible; human values must decide which tradeoffs to accept.
- Ethical portfolio management requires an explicit commitment to equity, scientific freedom, and long-term thinking, values that metrics-driven optimization may inadvertently undermine.

- Successful implementation needs step-by-step change management, stakeholder involvement, and ongoing monitoring and adjustments.

QUESTIONS FOR REFLECTION

1. How well does your institution's research portfolio align with its stated strategic priorities, and how might systematic analysis uncover gaps or misalignments?
2. What is the right balance between high-risk innovation and steady progress for your organization, and is that balance currently being achieved?
3. How could your institution better utilize its unique research strengths or tackle major capability gaps?
4. What ethical considerations should be prioritized in research portfolio decisions at your institution?
5. How can portfolio decisions be made more transparent and participatory while staying strategically coherent?
6. If AI indicates that your institution's portfolio is suboptimal based on certain metrics, how would you balance that analysis with the judgment of experienced research leaders?

NOTES

1. Fortunato, S., et al. (2018). Science of science. *Science*, 359(6379), eaao0185. https://doi.org/10.1126/science.aao0185. Note: This comprehensive review covers computational approaches to understanding research dynamics, including publication trends, citation networks, collaboration patterns, and the prediction of scientific impact, the intellectual foundation for AI-powered environmental scanning and portfolio analysis.
2. Markowitz, H. (1952). Portfolio selection. *Journal of Finance*, 7(1), 77–91. https://doi.org/10.2307/2975974. Note: The foundational paper on portfolio diversification theory. While developed for financial portfolios, the core insight that diversification across imperfectly correlated assets reduces risk has been adapted to research portfolio contexts, though with important limitations discussed in this chapter.

3. Belton, V., & Stewart, T. J. (2002). *Multiple Criteria Decision Analysis: An Integrated Approach*. Kluwer Academic Publishers.
4. Wang, D., Song, C., & Barabási, A. L. (2013). Quantifying long-term scientific impact. *Science*, 342, 127–132. https://doi.org/10.1126/science.1237825
5. Packalen, M., & Bhattacharya, J. (2020). NIH funding and the pursuit of edge science. *Proceedings of the National Academy of Sciences*, 117(22), 12011–12016. https://doi.org/10.1073/pnas.1910160117. Note: This study directly examines risk-return tradeoffs in research funding, finding that NIH-funded research has become increasingly conservative and less likely to build on novel scientific ideas, a finding with direct implications for portfolio risk management.
6. Uzzi, B., Mukherjee, S., Stringer, M., & Jones, B. (2013). Atypical combinations and scientific impact. *Science*, 342, 468–472. https://doi.org/10.1126/science.1240474
7. Burt, R. S. (2004). Structural holes and good ideas. *American Journal of Sociology*, 110(2), 349–399. https://doi.org/10.1086/421787
8. Moed, H. F. (2005). *Citation Analysis in Research Evaluation*. Springer.

7 AI for Team Assembly and Collaboration

THE CHALLENGE OF RESEARCH COLLABORATION

Research has shifted from a mostly solitary activity to a more collaborative one. An analysis of 19.9 million papers over 50 years shows that teams are increasingly surpassing individual authors in producing knowledge, with team-authored papers not only becoming more common but also earning more citations, a trend that has grown over time.[1] Even in mathematics, once seen as the realm of lone thinkers, the share of team-produced work increased from 19% to 57% during the study period. This change reflects the growing complexity of research questions, the interdisciplinary nature of many key problems, and the specialized expertise needed to use advanced methods.

Building effective research teams remains remarkably challenging. Finding researchers with complementary skills, compatible working styles, and shared interests largely depends on existing networks, conference interactions, and colleague recommendations, channels that can overlook ideal collaborators working in different circles or institutions. Once potential partners are identified, assembling a strong team involves balancing complementary expertise with communication needs, diversity of perspectives with shared language, and team size with coordination complexity. These challenges increase when collaborations extend across institutions, countries, or the divide between academic research and community engagement.

Artificial intelligence (AI) can assist in tackling some of these challenges by analyzing expertise patterns on a large

 DOI 10.1201/9781003782995-10

scale, mapping collaboration networks that would be invisible to individual researchers, identifying potential partners based on complementary skills rather than just proximity, and flagging issues, from skill gaps to conflicts of interest, that need human attention. However, successful collaborations ultimately depend on human relationships, trust, communication, and shared commitment. AI can suggest who might be a good collaborator; it cannot make the collaboration succeed. This chapter discusses where AI truly adds value in building teams and where human judgment remains crucial.

IDENTIFYING COINVESTIGATORS AND COLLABORATORS

The first step in forming research teams is to identify potential collaborators with relevant expertise and complementary skills. This is an area where AI's capacity to process large amounts of information offers a real advantage over traditional methods.

EXPERTISE PROFILING

AI can create detailed profiles of researchers' expertise that go far beyond what any CV or departmental webpage presents. By analyzing publication records with natural language processing, AI can gain a nuanced understanding of research topics, methods, and contributions, not just through simple keyword matching but through semantic analysis that recognizes conceptual relationships across different terminologies and disciplinary conventions.[2] Citation patterns show which parts of a researcher's work attract the most attention, indicating areas of unique influence. Grant portfolios highlight active research programs and proven capabilities. Collaboration histories reveal not only who researchers have worked with but also what roles they've played in team projects and whether those collaborations have been productive. Additionally, temporal analysis tracks how expertise develops over time, pinpointing emerging interests and new skills that a static profile might miss.

These profiles become powerful when combined with semantic matching that identifies researchers working on conceptually related problems even when they use entirely different language. A psychologist studying "cognitive load in decision-making" and a computer scientist researching "information overload in human-computer interaction" may be natural collaborators despite never appearing in each other's keyword searches. AI concept mapping can recognize these connections, identify methodological bridges where one researcher's techniques could be productively applied to another's questions, and surface complementary approaches, researchers studying different facets of related phenomena whose integration might yield insights neither could achieve alone.

NETWORK-BASED DISCOVERY

Analyzing collaboration networks uncovers potential partners through structural patterns, not just topical similarity. The idea that weak ties, connections through acquaintances rather than close colleagues, more often link separate communities suggests that some of the most valuable new collaborators may be found not among one's close contacts but among their contacts' contacts.[3] AI can systematically find these second-degree connections, evaluate their relevance, and identify researchers who connect otherwise separate research groups and could act as collaboration catalysts.

Beyond individual connections, AI can recognize entire research communities working on related topics through separate networks, parallel worlds of scholarship exploring similar questions from different perspectives, unaware of each other's progress. These disconnections highlight both inefficiencies and opportunities: linking them could prevent duplicate efforts and inspire integrative insights that neither community could achieve alone.

Practical constraints inevitably influence the feasibility of collaboration. Geographic proximity still matters when face-to-face interaction is essential, and AI can incorporate this into recommendations. Institutional compatibility, such as whether potential partners' institutions share similar research cultures, administrative processes, and collaboration histories, affects whether a scientifically promising partnership can function effectively. Resource complementarity or identifying partners at institutions with facilities or data that complement one's own can make collaborations more productive than the sum of their parts. For international collaborations, time zone alignment impacts whether teams can communicate synchronously, a factor that is more important for some working styles than others.

EXPERTISE MATCHING AND TEAM COMPOSITION

Identifying potential collaborators is just the start. Forming an effective team involves evaluating whether a specific group of researchers offers the right combination of skills, perspectives, and working styles.

COMPLEMENTARITY AND COVERAGE

Effective teams are made up of complementary rather than redundant expertise. AI can conduct systematic skill gap analysis, comparing a team's collective abilities to the requirements of a research project and pinpointing missing key expertise. It can identify excessive overlap, where team members have almost identical skills, indicating that one position might be better filled by someone with different capabilities. Additionally, it can assess methodological balance to ensure the team has the right mix of theoretical, methodological, and applied expertise instead of clustering in just one area.

Team size is a deceptively important decision. Research on scientific teams consistently shows a complex relationship between size and outcomes: larger teams tend to produce higher-impact work as measured by citations, but the relationship between team size and genuine novelty follows an inverted-U curve, with moderate-sized teams generating the most novel contributions.[1,4] This pattern likely reflects the tension between the information-processing advantages of larger groups and the coordination costs that grow with team size. AI can help researchers navigate this tension by analyzing what team sizes have been most productive for similar research projects in their field and estimating the minimum viable team, the smallest group that possesses all necessary expertise, as a starting point for team construction.

COLLABORATIVE FIT

Beyond credentials, whether potential collaborators will work well together is crucial and much harder to evaluate using algorithms. AI can assess whether potential team members have collaborated successfully before, if they share compatible approaches to authorship and data sharing, and if their communication styles (responsiveness, clarity, and engagement) indicate compatibility. However, these signals are noisy indicators of the interpersonal chemistry that actually determines whether a collaboration succeeds or struggles. The limitations section of this chapter directly addresses this challenge.

DIVERSITY AND INCLUSION IN TEAM BUILDING

Research teams gain from diverse perspectives, and building inclusive teams is both ethically crucial and scientifically effective. Evidence indicates that teams combining conventional and unconventional knowledge, drawing on unexpected combinations of prior work, produce more impactful science, and that teams spanning different fields and task types make more novel contributions.[4,5] These results provide an empirical basis for the idea that diversity matters, while also clarifying which types of diversity are most important for specific outcomes.

THE MULTIDIMENSIONAL NATURE OF RESEARCH DIVERSITY

Diversity in research teams is multidimensional and functionally essential for innovation. Disciplinary diversity introduces diverse theoretical frameworks and methodological approaches, generating integrative insights that no single discipline could produce. Demographic diversity, including gender, race, ethnicity, and background, provides varied lived experiences and perspectives that help prevent blind spots in research design and interpretation. Notably, research into the "diversity-innovation paradox" suggests that historically underrepresented groups produce higher rates of scientific novelty by introducing unconventional conceptual linkages that their peers might overlook.[6]

Career stage diversity combines the deep expertise and institutional knowledge of seasoned researchers with the fresh viewpoints and current technical skills of early-career investigators. Geographic and institutional diversity add critical contextual knowledge, while cognitive diversity, differences in mental models and problem-solving heuristics, serves as a primary driver of "collective intelligence." Theoretical modeling and empirical studies demonstrate that cognitively diverse groups consistently outperform homogeneous groups of high-ability individuals when solving the complex, nonroutine problems that characterize modern biomedical research.[7,8]

THE CHALLENGE OF SYSTEMIC HOMOPHILY

The challenge is that traditional networking patterns often reinforce existing inequalities. Opportunities for collaboration tend to go through established networks that may systematically exclude talented researchers from less privileged backgrounds, institutions, or demographic groups. Homophily, the well-documented tendency in science to collaborate with similar others, creates "echo chambers" of thought that stifle the very cognitive diversity required for breakthrough discovery.

Without intentional intervention, AI recommendation systems trained on historical collaboration data will tend to reproduce rather than challenge existing inequalities. Because these models are trained on the scholarly past, they risk inadvertently scaling the "Matthew Effect," a phenomenon first described by Robert Merton (1968) where eminent scientists receive disproportionately more credit than less-famous researchers for similar work.[9] In the age of generative AI, this "cumulative advantage" is amplified at scale, as algorithms prioritize already-prominent "hubs" in the scientific network, potentially marginalizing the diverse perspectives necessary to move science from incrementalism to transformation.[10,11]

THE MATILDA EFFECT: GENDERED BIAS IN SCIENTIFIC ATTRIBUTION

While the Matthew Effect describes the general cumulative advantage of elite researchers, demographic diversity in science is further compromised by the "Matilda Effect." Coined by historian Margaret W. Rossiter (1993), the Matilda Effect describes the systematic underrecognition of the contributions of female scientists, whose work is often attributed to their male colleagues or downplayed in historical records. This phenomenon is particularly relevant in the history of biomedical discovery, where women's roles in foundational breakthroughs, from the structure of DNA to the development of early vaccines, were frequently obscured or credited to male laboratory heads.[12,13]

In the context of AI-driven research, the Matilda Effect poses a significant risk to the integrity of automated discovery. If AI discovery tools and "expertise-mapping" algorithms are trained on historical publication and citation data that reflect these gendered biases, they will naturally "learn" to undervalue the expertise of female researchers. This creates a recursive loop of exclusion:

- **Algorithmic Erasure**: AI models may fail to identify female investigators as "experts" or "key opinion leaders" because their citation counts have been suppressed by historical attribution bias.
- **Recommendation Feedback Loops**: When AI suggests potential collaborators or guest speakers, it may favor male researchers who have benefited from the Matthew Effect, thereby scaling the Matilda Effect into the digital future.

- **Impact Assessment Bias**: Automated systems used by tenure committees or funding agencies to evaluate "research impact" may provide lower scores to women if the training data does not account for the structural undercitation of female-led work.[14]

BIAS DETECTION AND INCLUSIVE RECOMMENDATION

AI can play a constructive role by making collaboration biases visible and helping to correct them. Homophily detection can reveal when collaboration networks are excessively homogeneous. Structural inequality identification can show when certain groups are systematically excluded from central network positions. Opportunity gap analysis can identify talented researchers from underrepresented groups who lack collaboration opportunities despite having relevant expertise.

Critically, inclusive recommendation systems must do more than passively avoid bias; they should also actively promote qualified researchers from underrepresented groups. This involves regularly auditing recommendation algorithms for bias, intentionally suggesting network expansions that help researchers diversify beyond current patterns, and identifying structural barriers, not just individual biases, that hinder certain researchers' collaboration opportunities. Equitable partnership assessment can evaluate whether authorship patterns, resource distribution, and decision-making power are fairly shared within existing collaborations, providing feedback to help teams recognize and address internal inequalities.

CONFLICT OF INTEREST DETECTION

Research collaborations must identify and manage conflicts of interest, financial, personal, or professional relationships that could compromise research objectivity. This is an area where AI's ability to systematically cross-reference multiple data sources provides practical value.

AI can analyze funding sources to identify when team members have financial relationships with relevant entities, scan patent and equity databases for intellectual property stakes that could create conflicts, and flag consulting relationships or institutional financial interests that might compromise objectivity. Personal relationship conflicts, family ties, supervisory relationships, and close personal connections are harder to detect algorithmically but can sometimes be identified through coauthorship patterns, shared institutional histories, or disclosed relationships in public databases.

Professional conflicts require special attention. Competitive relationships between potential collaborators, histories of disputes, and situations where team members might inappropriately review each other's work can all weaken collaboration. AI can identify these risks, but managing them depends on human judgment: assessing whether a conflict is significant, developing suitable management plans, setting recusal protocols when needed, and establishing oversight systems to ensure conflicts do not compromise research integrity.

The goal is not to eliminate all potential conflicts, which would hinder collaboration, but to identify, disclose, and manage relevant conflicts properly before they cause issues.

CROSS-INSTITUTIONAL AND INTERNATIONAL PARTNERSHIPS

Collaborations across institutions and countries present great scientific opportunities but involve managing logistical, administrative, cultural, and regulatory challenges that single-institution research does not face.

INSTITUTIONAL PARTNERSHIP ASSESSMENT

AI can assess institutional compatibility across key dimensions for successful collaboration. Historical patterns of collaboration between institutions show whether their administrative processes have worked well together. Resource complementarity analysis determines how different institutions' facilities, equipment, and data assets enhance each other, making the partnership stronger than either could be alone. Additionally, if research cultures can be characterized by publication patterns, collaboration norms, and institutional policies, AI can identify potential friction points before they turn into issues.

INTERNATIONAL COLLABORATION

Global partnerships add layers of complexity that require careful navigation. Different countries maintain different research regulations, ethics review requirements, data protection laws, and intellectual property frameworks.[15] AI can map this regulatory landscape, helping researchers understand requirements before committing to partnerships. Identifying multilingual researchers who can serve as cultural brokers, navigating not just language differences but divergent research norms and expectations, is valuable for collaborations spanning cultural contexts. Practical considerations like time zone optimization, while seemingly minor, significantly affect whether distributed teams can maintain the synchronous communication many collaborations require.

Partnership sustainability is a crucial issue, especially in international collaborations where power imbalances between institutions are common. AI can evaluate whether proposed partnerships benefit all parties equally rather than just providing extractive value in one direction, identify chances for real capacity building at each partner institution, and determine if knowledge exchange is bidirectional. These evaluations need human interpretation and ethical judgment, but AI can offer structured analysis that makes these conversations more concrete and accountable.

COMMUNITY AND PATIENT PARTNER IDENTIFICATION

For community-based and patient-centered research, it is crucial to identify and engage suitable partners beyond academic researchers, and this presents unique challenges that exceed traditional collaborator identification.

FINDING AND ENGAGING COMMUNITY PARTNERS

Community partnership requires understanding community structures, histories, and trust relationships that are largely invisible to the databases AI typically analyzes. AI can help map community organizations that represent relevant populations, identify patient advocacy organizations, and assess which organizations are actively engaged in research. But the most critical partnership questions, which organizations have genuine community trust and legitimacy, what historical relationships (positive or negative) exist between academic institutions and communities, and whether potential partners have both the interest and capacity for sustained research engagement, require human knowledge and relationship-building that AI cannot provide.

AI's most valuable contribution may be in supporting the design of equitable partnerships once partners are identified. Power balance assessment can evaluate whether partnerships are genuinely collaborative or whether academic partners maintain de facto control. Compensation analysis can ensure community and patient partners are appropriately recognized and compensated. Benefit-sharing frameworks can be assessed for equity. And coproduction approaches, structuring research as genuine collaboration rather than consultation, can be supported by tools that track participation in decision-making and ensure all partners have a meaningful voice.

Cultural competence and respect are fundamental to all community partnerships. Identifying team members who can navigate cultural differences, ensuring research teams understand and respect cultural protocols, providing appropriate language access, and recognizing that meaningful partnerships require significant time for relationship and trust building are all prerequisites that AI can identify, but humans must fulfill.

FACILITATING TEAM COMMUNICATION AND COORDINATION

Once teams are formed, AI can assist with ongoing collaboration efforts. This field is becoming more mature, with a growing ecosystem of AI-powered tools for team coordination, although most are created for business teams rather than research collaborations specifically.[16]

AI adds practical value in areas like scheduling optimization across multiple time zones, generating meeting agendas based on project status, tracking action items across meetings, and monitoring participation to flag team members who are consistently marginalized in discussions. Document collaboration benefits from AI-assisted version control, contribution tracking, consistency checks across sections written by different team members, and style harmonization, the same capabilities discussed in the grant writing context of Chapter 3.

Conflict detection is a more sensitive tool. AI can potentially spot patterns indicating emerging team tensions, such as decreased communication, more negativity in written exchanges, or withdrawal by specific team members, and alert team leaders before issues worsen. However, this kind of monitoring raises valid privacy and autonomy concerns that teams should discuss openly before adopting it.

COLLABORATION NETWORK ANALYSIS AND STRATEGY

Understanding the structure of collaboration networks helps inform strategic decisions about partnerships at both individual and institutional levels.

Network mapping uncovers researchers' roles, whether they are central, peripheral, or bridging, and identifies clusters of closely collaborating researchers that form distinct research communities.[3] Tracking the evolution shows how networks shift over time, revealing increasing connections, waning relationships, and emerging communities. Gap detection highlights disconnections between communities that could benefit from bridging, the "structural holes" whose presence often links to innovation and new ideas.[17]

Strategic network building leverages these insights to guide intentional decisions about collaboration. Instead of allowing networks to grow solely through chance and proximity, researchers can identify collaborations that strategically expand their networks, connect isolated communities, and boost overall diversity. AI can also analyze the relationship between collaboration patterns and research impact, exploring whether collaborative efforts yield greater influence than individual work in specific fields, identifying team sizes that produce the highest-impact research, and examining how different collaboration types (within-institution, cross-institution, and international) influence results.[18]

PRACTICAL IMPLEMENTATION STRATEGIES

Effective use of AI for team assembly involves intentionally combining algorithmic suggestions with human insight. AI is most useful for discovery, finding potential collaborators that researchers might not otherwise discover, and for analysis, evaluating team composition and spotting potential gaps or issues. Humans remain crucial for relationship building, creating trust and rapport that make collaborations successful, negotiation, navigating the interpersonal and institutional complexities of partnerships, and judgment, assessing whether a partnership that seems promising on paper will actually work given the specific people and contexts involved.

Privacy and consent need careful attention. Using AI to analyze researchers' publication records, collaboration histories, and expertise profiles for matching raises issues about data transparency, consent, profile accuracy, and recommendation clarity. Opt-in methods, allowing researchers to choose whether to participate in matching systems and review and correct their automatically generated profiles, respect autonomy while still enabling the benefits of AI discovery.

Validation is crucial and often overlooked. AI collaboration systems should be regularly evaluated for recommendation quality (do suggested collaborations actually prove productive?), bias (do algorithms systematically favor certain types of researchers?), and user satisfaction (do researchers find the recommendations useful and relevant?). Without this feedback loop, systems may optimize for the wrong goals or unknowingly reinforce biases.

CAPABILITIES AND LIMITATIONS: THE TEAM SCIENCE AUDIT

While the Master Matrix in Chapter 1 outlines general AI strengths in Pattern Analysis and Collaboration Support, applying these to team assembly requires a specialized set of Override Triggers. Building a research team is a sociological exercise, not just a talent-matching one. AI can map "expertise" based on existing data, but as discussed earlier in this chapter, that data is often poisoned by the Matilda Effect and historical attribution biases (Table 7.1).

TABLE 7.1
Collaboration-Specific Override Protocols

Assembly Task	AI Execution (The "Meat")	The Human Override (The Top Bread)
Expertise mapping	Analyzing publication records and grant histories to build researcher profiles	**Bias Audit:** AI mirrors the "Matthew Effect." The human must manually search for rising stars and underrecognized experts to counter **Algorithmic Erasure**
Network visualization	Mapping coauthorship networks to identify structural "holes" or opportunities	**Culture Check:** AI sees *connections*; humans see *conflicts*. Determine if a potential link is blocked by departmental politics or historical rivalries
Complementarity analysis	Evaluating whether team members offer redundant or unique skill sets	**Soft-Skill Appraisal:** AI assesses *CVs*; humans must assess *personalities*. A redundant skill set is often better than a "perfect" technical match with a toxic work style

(*Continued*)

TABLE 7.1 (*Continued*)
Collaboration-Specific Override Protocols

Assembly Task	AI Execution (The "Meat")	The Human Override (The Top Bread)
Diversity auditing	Scanning team compositions for demographic and disciplinary balance	**Innovation Check:** Guard against "tokenism." Ensure the AI isn't just optimizing for keywords but is supporting the **Innovation-Diversity Paradox** through genuine inclusion

Refer to the Master Matrix in Chapter 1 for foundational failure modes; the table outlines the expert-level interventions required for team assembly.

NEUTRALIZING THE MATILDA EFFECT IN RECOMMENDATIONS

As detailed in our previous discussion of Algorithmic Erasure, AI models are trained on historical citation data that systematically undervalues female investigators. In the "Execution" phase of team assembly, the AI will naturally favor male researchers who have benefited from the Matthew Effect.

- **The AI Limit**: AI optimizes for "proven impact," which is often a proxy for historical privilege rather than future potential.
- **The Human Task**: You must trigger an Equity Intervention. When the AI suggests potential collaborators or "key opinion leaders," the human investigator must intentionally scout for the female and underrepresented researchers the algorithm has deprioritized. Use the AI to find the "obvious" names and then use your professional network to find the "erased" experts.

CHEMISTRY, TRUST, AND THE "INNOVATION-DIVERSITY PARADOX"

Effective collaboration depends on human connection, a variable that remains invisible to AI:

1. **Trust versus Reliability**: AI can track if a collaborator meets deadlines, but it cannot evaluate *trustworthiness*, the shared commitment to ethical conduct and intellectual honesty.
2. **Conflict Prediction**: AI can detect a conflict once it is recorded in text (e.g., in emails), but it cannot *foresee* a mismatch in working styles or underlying motivations before the project begins.
3. **The Paradox of Diversity**: While diverse teams are more innovative, they often face higher initial friction. AI often optimizes for "seamless" coordination, which can inadvertently lead to "groupthink" by suggesting collaborators who are too similar to the Principal Investigator.

The Override Trigger: If the AI suggests a "perfect" team on paper that lacks interpersonal history or diversity of thought, you must trigger a Chemistry Interview. You are the final judge of who will stand by the project during a clinical crisis; the AI is merely a matchmaker of technical credentials.

THE SKEPTIC'S CORNER

- **Target Task**: Expertise mapping and team composition.
- **Adversarial Prompt**: "Evaluate the proposed research team for [Project]. Identify potential groupthink risks given their shared institutional histories, and list three critical gaps in technical expertise that this team structure currently overlooks."

ETHICAL CONSIDERATIONS

Using AI for team assembly raises ethical concerns that require clear attention. Reproducing historical bias is likely the most significant issue: systems trained on past collaboration patterns tend to suggest familiar partnerships, which can reinforce existing inequalities and exclusions. Bias in metrics makes this worse; relying on easy-to-quantify indicators like publications and citations can unfairly disadvantage researchers with less conventional but valuable expertise, such as community partners, clinical practitioners, and early-career investigators. Network privilege also plays a role; researchers already in central positions in the network get more recommendations, deepening existing advantages.

Fairness requires active effort, not just neutrality. Recommendation systems should be regularly checked for demographic bias and designed to encourage inclusive team building, rather than merely to avoid blatant discrimination. At the same time, researcher autonomy must be maintained: AI should suggest rather than dictate collaborations, researchers should be able to decline recommendations without penalty, and the reasoning behind specific suggestions should be transparent and explainable.

Privacy concerns are valid. Analyzing researchers' professional activities for matching purposes, even when only using publicly available data, can create profiles that researchers might not want generated or shared. Clear policies on data sources, purposes, and researcher control over their profiles are vital for maintaining trust in these systems.

LOOKING FORWARD

AI capabilities for supporting collaboration continue to advance on multiple fronts. Improved matching algorithms now incorporate a deeper understanding of expertise, compatibility, and complementarity, going beyond just simple topical overlap. Real-time collaboration support systems are evolving from initial matching to continuous facilitation, helping teams maintain effective communication, resolve conflicts, and coordinate tasks throughout a project's duration. Virtual collaboration tools are becoming more advanced, offering better support for the distributed teams that increasingly characterize modern research. Additionally, inclusive network-building approaches are gaining more attention, with systems designed to expand rather than reinforce existing collaboration patterns.

However, the core nature of research collaboration, building trusting relationships and working effectively with others toward common goals, will remain fundamentally human work. The most promising direction is not AI replacing human judgment about collaboration, but rather AI broadening the pool of potential collaborators researchers can identify and evaluate, while humans maintain complete authority over the relationship decisions that influence collaboration success.

CONCLUSION

Modern research increasingly demands collaboration across disciplines, institutions, and sectors, and AI provides powerful tools to facilitate team formation: identifying potential collaborators among large researcher populations, evaluating team composition for complementarity and gaps, promoting diversity and inclusion, detecting conflicts of interest, and managing partnership logistics. These capabilities enable researchers to find partners they might not otherwise encounter and to assemble teams with the diverse expertise needed for complex research challenges.

Successful collaboration, however, ultimately relies on human relationships, trust, communication, and shared commitment, elements that AI cannot reliably create or evaluate. The most effective approach combines AI's analytical abilities for discovery and assessment with human skills for relationship building, interpersonal evaluation, and maintaining the trust that keeps partnerships strong. When used thoughtfully and ethically, AI for team assembly can help ensure research teams include the diverse expertise and perspectives needed to answer important questions, while also fostering more inclusive and equitable collaboration patterns.

The next chapter examines how AI can aid in research administration and compliance, assisting organizations in navigating the complicated regulatory and administrative requirements that oversee research conduct.

KEY TAKEAWAYS

- Team-authored research has become dominant across disciplines and generates higher-impact work, making team assembly an ever more important research skill.
- AI can identify potential collaborators by semantically analyzing expertise profiles, mapping collaboration networks, and recognizing complementary capabilities across disciplinary boundaries.
- Effective team composition involves balancing complementary expertise, selecting an appropriate team size (with evidence suggesting that moderate-sized teams produce the most innovative work), defining clear roles, and ensuring collaborative compatibility.
- Building diverse and inclusive teams demands intentional effort to counteract homophily; AI recommendation systems should be designed to actively foster inclusion instead of perpetuating existing biases.
- Conflict of interest detection benefits from AI's ability to cross-reference financial, personal, and professional relationships across multiple databases.
- Cross-institutional and international partnerships require AI analysis of compatibility combined with significant human effort in cultural understanding and relationship development.
- Community and patient partnerships require approaches that ensure equity, respect, and true coproduction, areas where AI can assist with assessment, but humans must lead engagement.
- Interpersonal chemistry, trust, motivation alignment, and conflict prediction remain beyond AI's abilities, making human judgment crucial for all final collaboration decisions.

QUESTIONS FOR REFLECTION

1. How can AI-supported collaborator discovery assist you in finding partners beyond your current network who could enhance your research?

2. What aspects of diversity are most important for your research teams, and how might you intentionally foster more diverse collaborations?
3. How can you make sure AI-suggested collaborations result in fair partnerships instead of exploitative ones?
4. What potential conflicts of interest should you be especially aware of in your collaborative work?
5. How can you more effectively bring community and patient partners into your research teams as true collaborators instead of just consultants?
6. What would you want to learn about a potential collaborator that AI can't tell you, and how would you discover it?

NOTES

1. Wuchty, S., Jones, B. F., & Uzzi, B. (2007). The increasing dominance of teams in production of knowledge. *Science*, 316, 1036–1039. https://doi.org/10.1126/science.1136099
2. Fortunato, S., et al. (2018). Science of science. *Science*, 359, eaao0185. https://doi.org/10.1126/science.aao0185. Note: This comprehensive review covers computational approaches to analyzing expertise, collaboration networks, and research dynamics, the analytical foundation for AI-powered collaborator identification systems.
3. Granovetter, M. S. (1973). The strength of weak ties. *American Journal of Sociology*, 78(6), 1360–1380. https://doi.org/10.1086/225469. Note: Granovetter's foundational insight that weak ties bridge otherwise disconnected communities underpins network-based collaborator discovery. Second-degree connections and structural bridges are particularly valuable for identifying collaborators outside existing networks.
4. Lee, Y. N., Walsh, J. P., & Wang, J. (2015). Creativity in scientific teams: Unpacking novelty and impact. *Research Policy*, 44(3), 684–697. https://doi.org/10.1016/j.respol.2014.10.007. Note: This study found an inverted-U relationship between team size and novelty, with team field and task variety largely explaining this pattern, while team size had a continually increasing relationship with likelihood of high-impact work.
5. Uzzi, B., Mukherjee, S., Stringer, M., & Jones, B. (2013). Atypical combinations and scientific impact. *Science*, 342, 468–472. https://doi.org/10.1126/science.1240474. Note: This study found

that the highest-impact papers combine predominantly conventional knowledge with an injection of atypical, novel combinations, a finding that supports the value of teams spanning different knowledge domains, though the paper analyzes knowledge combinations rather than team diversity per se.

6. Hofstra, B., et al. (2020). The diversity–innovation paradox in science. *Proceedings of the National Academy of Sciences (PNAS)*, 117(17), 9284–9291.
7. Page, S. E. (2007). *The Difference: How the Power of Diversity Creates Better Groups, Firms, Schools, and Societies*. Princeton University Press.
8. Woolley, A. W., et al. (2010). Evidence for a collective intelligence factor in the performance of human groups. *Science*, 330, 686–688. https://doi.org/10.1126/science.1193147
9. Merton, R. K. (1968). The Matthew effect in science: The reward and communication systems of science are considered. *Science*, 159(3810), 56–63. https://doi.org/10.1126/science.159.3810.56
10. Pooley, J. (2025). The Matthew effect in AI summary. *JeffPooley.com*. https://www.jeffpooley.com/2025/11/the-matthew-effect-in-ai-summary/
11. Schrepel, T. (2024). The Matthew effect at scale: Attention scarcity and the AI output explosion. *Network Law Review*. https://www.networklawreview.org/matthew-effect/
12. Rossiter, M. W. (1993). The Matthew Matilda effect in science. *Social Studies of Science*, 23(2), 325–341. https://doi.org/10.1177/030631293023002004
13. Lincoln, A. E., Pincus, S., Koster, J. B., & Leboy, P. S. (2012). The Matilda effect in science: Awards and prizes in the US, 1990s and 2000s. *Social Studies of Science*, 42(2), 307–320. https://doi.org/10.1177/0306312711435830
14. Larivière, V., Ni, C., Gingras, Y., Cronin, B., & Sugimoto, C. R. (2013). Bibliometrics: Global gender disparities in science. *Nature*, 504(7479), 211–213. https://doi.org/10.1038/504211a
15. Anderson, M., & Stenbeck, N. (2011). *International Research Collaborations: Much to Be Gained, Many Ways to Get in Trouble*. Taylor & Francis. https://doi.org/10.4324/9780203848906
16. Vibe.us. (2026, January 8). 19 AI collaboration tools for innovative teams in 2026. https://vibe.us/blog/top-collaboration-tools-for-remote-teams/. Note: Representative of the rapidly growing ecosystem of AI-powered collaboration tools. While most are designed for business teams, their scheduling, document collaboration, and communication features are increasingly applicable to research team coordination.

17. Burt, R. S. (2004). Structural holes and good ideas. *American Journal of Sociology*, 110(2), 349–399. https://doi.org/10.1086/421787. Note: Burt's research demonstrates that individuals bridging "structural holes," gaps between otherwise disconnected network clusters, generate more good ideas, a finding with direct implications for strategic collaboration network building.
18. Wu, L., Wang, D., & Evans, J. A. (2019). Large teams develop and small teams disrupt science and technology. *Nature*, 566, 378–382. https://doi.org/10.1038/s41586-019-0941-9. Note: This study of 65 million papers, patents, and software products found that small teams tend to produce disruptive, novel work while large teams tend to develop existing ideas, a finding that informs optimal team size decisions and portfolio-level thinking about team composition.

8 AI for Biomedical Research Administration and Compliance

THE CHALLENGE OF RESEARCH ADMINISTRATION AND COMPLIANCE

Research administration involves navigating a complex landscape of overlapping regulatory frameworks, which would challenge even the most dedicated compliance professional. Federal regulations, including the Common Rule for human subjects research, FDA rules for drugs and devices, and HIPAA for health information privacy, are layered on top of state laws, institutional policies, international regulations for cross-border collaborations, and funder-specific requirements. Knowing which frameworks apply to a specific project and how they interact requires specialized expertise, something many institutions struggle to maintain at sufficient depth and scale.

The challenge starts with definitional confusion. Terms like "research" and "human subject" have regulatory definitions that don't always match everyday usage, and the lines between research, quality improvement (QI), program evaluation, and public health surveillance can be truly fuzzy. When different administrators interpret these definitions differently, similar projects get different rulings, causing inconsistency that confuses researchers and erodes trust in the system. Resource limits make it worse: research administrators are often overwhelmed by the high number of protocols needing review and

 DOI 10.1201/9781003782995-11

monitoring, with limited staff managing increasingly complex regulations. Documentation needs are extensive, including protocols, consent forms, data management plans, conflict of interest disclosures, progress reports, and regulations that change constantly, requiring continuous attention to stay up to date.

Multiinstitutional research adds another layer of complexity. Studies spanning multiple sites must navigate different institutional policies and procedures while ensuring all locations meet the necessary requirements, a coordination challenge that increases with the number of participating institutions. International collaborations introduce even more variables: diverse countries' research regulations, ethics review requirements, data protection laws, and export control considerations all require attention.

Artificial intelligence (AI) has real potential to solve some of these challenges by systematically analyzing regulatory requirements, applying criteria consistently, automating compliance checks, and managing documentation efficiently. However, compliance ultimately depends on human judgment to interpret how regulations apply to specific situations and determine if proposed research meets ethical standards. The most effective uses of AI are those where it manages the rule-based aspects of compliance and flags complex or unclear cases for human experts, enhancing administrative capacity without replacing human judgment.

DECISION SUPPORT FOR RESEARCH DETERMINATIONS

One of the most basic questions in research administration is whether planned activities qualify as "research" under federal regulations. Incorrectly making this determination can have impacts in either direction: activities labeled as nonresearch that should have been reviewed might go forward without proper oversight, while activities labeled as research that aren't could face unnecessary delays and administrative burdens.

THE DEFINITION CHALLENGE

The Common Rule defines research as "a systematic investigation, including research development, testing, and evaluation, designed to develop or contribute to generalizable knowledge."[1] This definition, while clear in principle, proves ambiguous in application. QI projects systematically collect and analyze data to improve local processes; program evaluations assess whether programs achieve intended outcomes; public health surveillance monitors population health indicators. Each shares characteristics with research but may not meet the regulatory definition, and the boundaries shift depending on intent, design, and dissemination plans.

AI can support these determinations in several ways that add genuine value. Structured decision support guides users through systematic questions about proposed activities, ensuring all relevant factors are considered rather than relying on whatever aspects happen to come to mind. Definitional analysis compares activity descriptions against regulatory criteria, identifying alignment or misalignment with key elements. Precedent matching, comparing proposed activities to a database of previous determinations, identifies similar cases and how they were classified, promoting consistency over time. And uncertainty flagging identifies borderline cases where characteristics suggest genuinely ambiguous classification, directing enhanced review to the cases that most need it rather than distributing review effort equally across easy and hard cases.

HUMAN SUBJECTS RESEARCH AND EXEMPTION DETERMINATIONS

Once an activity is determined to be research, the next question is whether it involves "human subjects," defined in the revised Common Rule based on whether investigators obtain information through intervention or interaction with individuals or obtain identifiable private information.[1] AI can analyze whether planned activities involve interactions meeting regulatory definitions, evaluate whether data sources contain identifiable private information, assess whether proposed deidentification approaches meet regulatory standards, and determine whether research might qualify for exempt status under specific exemption categories.[2]

The exemption determination is particularly well-suited to AI support because it involves matching study characteristics against defined criteria, a systematic task where consistency matters and where human reviewers sometimes apply criteria inconsistently. At the same time, exemption categories contain nuances and conditional requirements that demand careful reading, and certain categories (particularly those involving benign behavioral interventions or secondary use of identifiable information) require judgment about risk levels that AI should flag rather than resolve independently.

QI AND PROGRAM EVALUATION DISTINCTIONS

The boundary between QI and research is among the most contested in research administration. Both involve systematic investigation to improve outcomes, but QI focuses on improving local processes while research aims to generate generalizable knowledge. In practice, many projects share characteristics of both, and the distinction often turns on intent and design features that can be difficult to classify definitively.

AI can analyze whether activities are designed primarily to generate generalizable knowledge or improve local processes, whether findings will be disseminated beyond the local institution, whether methods prioritize rapid improvement cycles or rigorous knowledge generation, and whether the risk profile exceeds what participants would encounter in routine care or program participation. However, the QI/research distinction frequently requires nuanced judgment about investigator intent and project evolution, a QI project may generate findings worth publishing, at which point its classification may need reconsideration. AI serves best by ensuring systematic consideration of relevant factors while flagging genuinely ambiguous cases for human deliberation rather than forcing binary classifications where the underlying reality is a spectrum.

REGULATORY PATHWAY IDENTIFICATION

Once research is identified, determining the appropriate regulatory pathway is essential, and the options are numerous, with different requirements, timelines, and implications.

INSTITUTIONAL REVIEW BOARD (IRB) REVIEW CATEGORIES

Research involving human subjects requires IRB review, but several distinct pathways exist depending on risk level and study characteristics. Exempt research, qualifying under specific categories defined in the revised Common Rule, doesn't require continuing review after initial determination, though limited IRB review may still be required for certain categories.[2] Expedited review applies to research involving no more than minimal risk that fits specified categories, allowing review by a single experienced reviewer rather than the full board. Full board review is required for research that doesn't qualify for exemption or expedited review, typically studies involving more than minimal risk or vulnerable populations. AI can help classify studies into these categories by analyzing protocol characteristics against regulatory criteria, improving consistency and reducing the time administrators spend on straightforward classifications while ensuring that studies requiring full board scrutiny receive it.

Organizations developing AI-supported decision systems should align with emerging governance frameworks. The NIST AI Risk Management Framework provides structure for establishing accountability and oversight for AI administrative tools, organized around four core functions: governance, mapping, measurement, and management of AI-related risks.[3] The Joint Commission and Coalition for Health AI (CHAI) jointly released the Responsible Use of AI in Healthcare framework in September 2025, offering healthcare-specific guidance on governance structures, data protection, performance monitoring, and bias mitigation that research institutions can adapt for their compliance operations.[4] These frameworks emphasize the importance of designated AI leadership, risk-based oversight, and clear policies governing AI use in administrative functions.

FDA AND HIPAA PATHWAYS

For research regulated by the FDA, pathway identification involves determining whether investigational new drug applications or investigational device exemptions are necessary, whether studies qualify for exemptions, and when humanitarian device provisions might apply. AI can analyze study characteristics against FDA regulatory criteria to spot likely pathways, though final decisions usually require FDA expertise and often involve direct FDA consultation.

Research using protected health information must adhere to HIPAA Privacy Rule requirements, determining when authorization is necessary, when a waiver of authorization is appropriate, when limited dataset provisions with data use agreements (DUAs) are sufficient, and whether proposed deidentification meets safe harbor or expert determination standards. AI can systematically apply HIPAA decision trees, but complex cases involving new data types or unusual access patterns benefit from privacy officer expertise.

MULTISITE RESEARCH PATHWAYS

Under revised Common Rule requirements, most federally funded multisite research must use a single IRB review, a mandate that simplifies certain aspects of oversight while introducing new coordination challenges. AI can identify exceptions where local review remains suitable, determine the necessary reliance agreement types, manage site-specific issues even under single IRB arrangements, and facilitate communication between relying institutions and reviewing IRBs that single IRB models require.

AUTOMATED CONTRACT AND AGREEMENT ANALYSIS

Research produces a vast number of contracts and agreements, including sponsored research agreements, material transfer agreements (MTAs), DUAs, confidentiality agreements, and subaward contracts, each of which requires review in accordance with institutional policies and regulations. This is one of the most straightforward uses of AI in research administration, well-suited to natural language processing capabilities.

CONTRACT ABSTRACTION AND RISK FLAGGING

AI can extract key terms from contracts, such as payment amounts, deliverable deadlines, intellectual property provisions, publication rights, and termination clauses, and present them in standardized formats that facilitate quick review. Even more valuable, it can identify potentially problematic provisions: unusual indemnification requirements, restrictive publication terms that might limit academic freedom, insufficient protection of institutional interests, or clauses incompatible with federal funding requirements. Compliance checks can confirm that contracts include necessary provisions, such as conflict of interest clauses, data use restrictions, and language protecting human subjects, and can spot inconsistencies when multiple related contracts should be aligned but are not.

SPECIALIZED AGREEMENT TYPES

MTAs regulate the transfer of research materials between institutions. AI can identify when standard forms, such as the Uniform Biological MTA or Simple Letter Agreement, are used versus custom agreements; detect deviations from standard terms that require attention; highlight restrictions on material use that researchers need to understand; and ensure MTAs do not unduly restrict publication rights.

DUAs regulate access to restricted data. AI can verify that DUAs include all necessary elements for HIPAA limited datasets or other restricted data types, identify use limitations that researchers must follow, extract security requirements, and monitor expiration dates for renewal. Confidentiality agreements safeguard sensitive information in research collaborations, and AI can analyze their scope, exclusions, permitted disclosures, and potential conflicts between confidentiality provisions and publication or regulatory requirements.

These contract analysis applications are among the safest AI uses in research administration because the documents are structured, requirements are clear, and human review of flagged issues offers a natural quality control layer.

COMPLIANCE CHECKING AND MONITORING

Ongoing compliance monitoring is vital for maintaining research integrity but is resource-intensive and usually reactive instead of proactive. AI can transition compliance oversight to a systematic, continuous process.

PROTOCOL AND CONSENT COMPLIANCE

AI can oversee whether research follows approved protocols by monitoring enrollment within set limits and inclusion/exclusion criteria, verifying procedures against approved methods, ensuring timeline adherence, and flagging deviations from protocols that need modification submissions before implementation. These monitoring functions detect issues earlier than traditional periodic reviews, when corrective actions are still feasible.

Informed consent analysis is a highly valuable application. The FDA finalized comprehensive guidance on informed consent in August 2023, updating requirements for IRBs, investigators, and sponsors regarding the consent process and documentation.[5] AI can verify that consent forms include all elements required by regulation and institutional policy, assess readability to ensure forms are written at appropriate levels for target populations, check consistency between consent forms and protocols regarding procedures, risks, and benefits, and track consent form versions to prevent the use of outdated documents. These systematic checks catch errors that might otherwise reach participants, serving as an administrative protection function.

ADVERSE EVENT AND REGULATORY SUBMISSION MONITORING

For interventional research, adverse event monitoring involves identifying events across multiple data sources, evaluating their seriousness based on regulatory definitions, supporting relatedness assessments, determining reporting requirements and timelines, and recognizing concerning patterns that might not be evident from individual reviews. AI's pattern recognition capabilities are especially useful for this last task: detecting signals that event rates are higher than expected or that a certain subgroup is disproportionately impacted requires systematic data integration across sources that AI excels at.

Regulatory submission tracking, which involves identifying necessary submissions, monitoring deadlines, verifying completeness, and tracking responses and follow-up, is another area where AI's systematic approach provides significant value by preventing missed deadlines and incomplete submissions that could lead to serious compliance issues.

CONFLICT OF INTEREST MANAGEMENT

Financial and other conflicts of interest must be identified, disclosed, and managed to preserve research objectivity. AI can assist with each step of this process.

For identification, AI can analyze financial disclosures to detect relationships with relevant entities to researchers' work, determine whether financial interests surpass significance thresholds that require disclosure and management, and map connections between disclosed interests and research projects where conflicts might arise. Institutional conflicts, where the institution itself has financial interests that could conflict with research objectivity, are often harder to identify than individual conflicts but are equally important.

Disclosure analysis benefits from AI's ability to verify completeness, check consistency within and across disclosures, detect changes requiring updated reporting, and categorize whether disclosed interests are actual conflicts needing management versus relationships that don't pose significant risk. When conflicts exist, AI can identify standard management strategies (disclosure to participants, independent monitoring, and recusal from specific decisions), specify relevant regulations or policies, plan monitoring activities, and generate detailed documentation.

Ongoing conflict monitoring, tracking whether management plans are being followed, detecting changing circumstances, sending renewal reminders, and identifying patterns suggesting systematic issues, is exactly the kind of continuous, systematic oversight that AI handles well and that human administrators find challenging to maintain consistently across large research portfolios.

EXPORT CONTROL AND TECHNOLOGY TRANSFER

Research involving certain technologies, international collaborators, or foreign nationals may be subject to export controls, regulations that have received heightened enforcement attention in recent years.

EXPORT CONTROL SCREENING

Export control laws limit the transfer of certain technologies and information to foreign individuals or countries. AI can analyze research activities to determine whether they involve controlled technologies under the International Traffic in Arms Regulations or Export Administration Regulations, identify when research teams include foreign nationals whose access to controlled technologies might trigger legal requirements, screen international collaborators against restricted party lists, assess whether research qualifies for the fundamental research exemption, and determine when export licenses are needed.

The "deemed export" concept, in which foreign nationals' access to controlled technology in the United States constitutes an export requiring authorization, is especially relevant to universities and research institutions with international researchers. AI can identify when foreign nationals' access to controlled information or equipment might require authorization and evaluate how visa status influences these requirements.

The Bureau of Industry and Security (BIS) has increased its engagement with academic institutions through its Academic Outreach Initiative, launched in 2022 and expanded through

2024 with compliance guidance that highlights common violations found through voluntary self-disclosures.[6,7] Typical issues include unauthorized deemed exports to foreign national researchers, failure to classify controlled biological materials, and insufficient screening of international collaborators. BIS's 2025 interim final rule, which introduces a 50% ownership threshold, automatically extending Entity List restrictions to companies primarily owned by listed entities, further expands the scope of export control diligence needed when research involves commercial partnerships.[8] AI-driven screening can help institutions stay compliant with these changing requirements at a scale that manual processes cannot achieve.

TECHNOLOGY TRANSFER SUPPORT

When research leads to inventions or intellectual property, technology transfer processes need invention disclosure support, initial prior art assessment, identification of licensing opportunities, and facilitation of material transfers involving proprietary materials. AI can assist in each of these tasks, but patent strategy and licensing negotiations require the kind of strategic judgment that remains a human responsibility.

MULTIINSTITUTIONAL COMPLIANCE COORDINATION

Research across multiple institutions requires coordination that is logistically challenging and error-prone without systematic support. Under single IRB arrangements, AI can assist in managing reliance agreements, tracking institution-specific requirements even during centralized review, facilitating communication between relying sites and reviewing IRBs, and keeping organized documentation across all sites.

Site-specific compliance tracking is essential because, even with centralized IRB review, individual sites still have their own compliance duties, including institutional signing authority, research committee approvals, and local regulatory requirements.

AI can identify the requirements that vary across sites compared to those managed centrally, monitor local approvals, and record approved variations in how research is conducted at different locations. Central monitoring across sites can expose compliance pattern differences that might signal issues; for instance, a site with significantly higher protocol deviation rates may require additional training or oversight.

EMERGING AI APPLICATIONS FOR RESEARCH ADMINISTRATION

The use of AI in research administration is quickly progressing, with several significant developments. Researchers have proposed creating application-specific large language models (LLMs) designed for IRB review, fine-tuned with IRB-related documents, past decision records, and local policies.[9] These systems could review submissions for completeness, spot ethical issues, generate initial assessments, and ensure consistency with previous committee decisions. A related perspective in *BMC Medical Ethics* also emphasized both the potential advantages and the risks of this approach, noting that submitting IRB applications to AI tools raises confidentiality concerns, especially when applications include sensitive participant data, unpublished research ideas, or proprietary methods.[10] Without clear contractual safeguards on data retention and usage, institutions cannot guarantee that uploaded content won't be stored by AI developers, used to train future models, or accessed by unauthorized individuals.

PRIM&R's 2026 webinar series, including "AI and the IRB: When Are We Ready to Push 'Approved'?" (January 2026) and the upcoming "AI in Action: Institutional Innovations Supporting IRB Review" (April 2026), reflects the field's active engagement with these questions, exploring data privacy, transparency, bias, and practical institutional approaches to AI-supported review.[11]

These emerging applications demonstrate both the path and the conflicts in AI-supported research administration: the efficiency improvements are genuine and potentially significant, but they must be balanced against privacy concerns, the risk of overreliance on automated decisions, and the need for transparency about how AI affects administrative choices.

PRACTICAL IMPLEMENTATION STRATEGIES

Effective use of AI in research administration requires maintaining human oversight as a fundamental, nonnegotiable element. AI-supported decisions should always be verified by humans, with the authority to override when circumstances justify bypassing the algorithmic recommendations. AI systems must be able to explain their decisions, so administrators and researchers understand why a specific classification was made instead of just accepting an opaque result. Escalation procedures should establish clear criteria for referring complex or unusual cases to senior administrators or committees, rather than managing them solely through standard AI-supported processes.

Consistency and flexibility must coexist. AI can guarantee uniform application of regulatory standards, applying the same criteria to similar protocols regardless of which administrator manages them or when the review takes place, while human judgment retains the flexibility to consider context. When exceptions to standard decisions are made, clear documentation of rationales helps build the precedent database, making future AI decisions more precise and nuanced.

Training and change management are essential for successful implementation. Administrators must understand how AI systems work, their limitations, and when to trust or override their outputs. Researchers need to know how to interact with AI-supported systems and what to expect from them. Policies should be updated to reflect AI's role in administrative processes, and regular evaluation is important to assess whether AI support improves consistency, efficiency, and safety, rather than assuming it does.

Professional organizations are beginning to address this training need directly. PRIM&R has developed a comprehensive portfolio of AI-focused education for research oversight professionals, including a three-session Hands-On Core Training on Artificial Intelligence (December 2025) covering AI prompting techniques for administrative tasks, compliance evaluation of AI outputs, knowledge management, and ethical integration of AI into research administration workflows.[11] Their December 2025 symposium, "Balancing Innovation and Ethics: Artificial Intelligence in Research," brought together experts on AI in study design, data integrity, participant protections, and decision-making, including sessions on synthetic data governance and AI-specific consent.[11] These programs signal that the research oversight community recognizes the urgency of building AI competency among the professionals who will be using and overseeing these tools. PRIM&R has also advocated publicly for clear ethical guidelines governing data used in AI research, submitting formal comments to NTIA in January 2025 calling for "clear and comprehensive guidance" on the use of pervasive data in AI development.[12]

Integration with existing systems, such as electronic IRB platforms, grant management systems, conflict of interest databases, and export control screening tools, determines whether AI support simplifies workflows or unnecessary complexity. The most successful implementations connect AI capabilities across administrative functions rather than using isolated tools for individual tasks.

CAPABILITIES AND LIMITATIONS: THE RESEARCH ADMINISTRATION AUDIT

While the Master Matrix in Chapter 1 outlines general AI strengths in Regulatory Mapping and Oversight Tasks, applying these to research administration requires a specific set of Override Triggers. Administration is not merely about enforcing rules; it is about the professional judgment required to apply those rules to novel scientific scenarios. AI can identify a "noncompliance" pattern, but it cannot navigate the "regulatory gray zones" that define cutting-edge biomedical research (Table 8.1).

TABLE 8.1
Administration-Specific Override Protocols

Administrative Task	AI Execution (The "Meat")	The Human Override (The Top Bread)
Regulatory tracking	Systematically identifying which federal (FDA/OHRP) or international (EU AI Act) regulations apply to a protocol	**Temporal Audit:** Manually verify against the latest "Notice of Proposed Rulemaking" or 2026 agency guidance. AI training data often lags behind the current fiscal year's enforcement priorities
Cross-protocol monitoring	Reviewing an institution's entire portfolio for systemic compliance patterns or "red flags"	**Contextual Interpretation:** AI identifies *statistical* outliers; humans must identify *clinical* justifications. Determine if a "delay" is a compliance failure or a necessary safety pause
Documentation generation	Creating required reports, records, and registration entries (e.g., ClinicalTrials.gov) from structured data	**Accuracy Sign-off:** As documented in our 25% error rate audit, AI-generated technical data requires a 1:1 check. Ensure the AI hasn't "hallucinated" a value in a mandatory reporting field
Policy analysis	Drafting institutional standard operating procedures (SOPs) based on federal benchmarks	**Cultural Adaptation:** AI drafts "textbook" SOPs; humans must tailor them to the specific institutional culture and resource limits of the local site

Refer to the Master Matrix in Chapter 1 for foundational failure modes; the table outlines the expert-level interventions required for institutional oversight.

THE "LITERALIST" TRAP AND REGULATORY INTENT

A critical limitation in AI-driven administration is Algorithmic Rigidity. AI models process the *text* of a regulation but lack an understanding of the *intent* behind the law.

- **The AI Limit**: AI may flag a minor administrative deviation as a major violation because it cannot perform a proportionality judgment. It lacks the "wisdom" to know when a requirement is appropriate to the actual risk involved.
- **The Human Task**: You must provide the Advocacy Intervention. Use AI to identify potential gaps but trigger a Manual Override to determine if the situation requires a formal consultation with a regulatory body or a streamlined approach based on low-risk status.

STAKEHOLDER EMPATHY AND NOVELTY GAPS

Research administration relies on communication and the management of "human variables" that remain invisible to AI:

1. **Navigating "Gaps"**: Genuinely innovative research often falls between existing regulatory categories. AI will attempt to "force-fit" a novel study into an old box; humans must recognize the ambiguity and negotiate a new path with stakeholders.
2. **Communicating "No"**: Explaining a compliance rejection or a required modification to a frustrated researcher requires empathy and the ability to suggest constructive solutions. AI-generated "rejection letters" are often tone-deaf and can damage the relationship between the administration and the scientific faculty.
3. **Cultural Sensitivity**: As research involves international collaborations, understanding how local cultural contexts influence consent and data practices requires human cultural competence. AI cannot "see" the social dynamics that determine whether a participant recruitment strategy is ethically sound in a specific community.

The Override Trigger: If the AI suggests a "literal" interpretation of a regulation that halts a low-risk study or ignores the clinical reality of a trial, you must trigger a Regulatory Consultation Bypass. You are the final arbiter of how protections are applied; the AI is merely a monitor of the established text.

THE SKEPTIC'S CORNER

- **Target Task**: Regulatory determinations and contract review.
- **Adversarial Prompt**: "You determined this project is 'Not Human Subjects Research'. Now, act as an auditor from the OHRP. Provide a rigorous argument for why this project actually requires Full Board Review under the revised Common Rule."

ETHICAL CONSIDERATIONS

Using AI for biomedical research administration raises ethical questions that reflect the technology's dual ability to enhance and potentially undermine research protections.

The primary concern is ensuring that efficiency improvements do not compromise safety. If AI enables administrators to handle more protocols, the key question is whether each protocol receives enough review, not just whether the total number processed has increased. Risk-appropriate review, making sure that higher-risk research undergoes more thorough evaluation while lower-risk protocols are processed more efficiently, should be integrated into AI-supported workflows rather than assumed.

Algorithmic bias is a real concern in administrative contexts. If AI learns from historical decisions, it may reproduce biases in how different types of research or researchers were treated. If past administrators were more likely to require full board review for community-based research than for laboratory studies with similar risk profiles, AI trained on those patterns will continue that disparity. Accessibility bias is also important to consider: AI systems that demand sophisticated interaction may disadvantage researchers less familiar with technology, potentially creating barriers for populations that already face obstacles in the research enterprise.

Transparency and accountability require that researchers understand why decisions are made, that strong appeal processes exist for AI-supported choices, that clear audit trails record the basis for administrative actions, and that policies explicitly specify which functions AI supports versus which require unmediated human judgment. Without these safeguards, AI-supported administration risks becoming a black box that researchers cannot effectively engage with or challenge.

LOOKING FORWARD

AI capabilities for research administration continue to advance across several promising areas. Improvements in natural language understanding will allow AI to better interpret protocols and research descriptions, reducing the need for strict structured formatting for accurate analysis. Predictive compliance, which identifies potential issues based on protocol features before problems occur, will enable more proactive rather than reactive management. Integrated workflows connecting AI support across all administrative tasks will reduce the fragmentation that currently exists in research compliance infrastructure. Real-time guidance systems providing interactive assistance as researchers develop protocols will identify issues during the design phase rather than at submission. Additionally, learning systems that improve through feedback while maintaining human oversight will become more accurate and context-aware over time.

However, the core nature of research administration, applying regulations and ethical principles to ensure research protects participants and maintains integrity, will remain fundamentally human work. The goal is not autonomous compliance but enhanced compliance: AI making human administrators more effective, more consistent, and better able to focus their expertise where it matters most.

CONCLUSION

Research administration and compliance involve navigating complex regulatory frameworks to protect participants, ensure integrity, and uphold public trust. AI provides valuable support across all administrative tasks: analyzing whether activities qualify as research, identifying suitable regulatory pathways, automating contract review, monitoring compliance continuously, managing conflicts of interest, and screening for export controls.

These capabilities can enhance consistency, efficiency, and thoroughness in research administration by catching errors earlier, applying criteria more consistently, and monitoring compliance more continuously than human efforts alone. However, they function best when combined with human expertise in regulatory interpretation, ethical reasoning, contextual judgment, and the interpersonal communication that makes compliance a collaborative rather than adversarial process. When used correctly, AI for research administration helps ensure that research adheres to proper protections while also reducing unnecessary burdens on both researchers and administrators.

The next chapter investigates how AI can assist in optimizing IRB and ethics review processes, focusing on specific applications within IRB activities and research oversight.

KEY TAKEAWAYS

- Research administration involves navigating complex, overlapping regulatory frameworks, the Common Rule, FDA regulations, HIPAA, state laws, institutional policies, and funder requirements, which present significant compliance challenges.
- AI can assist in research versus nonresearch and human subjects determinations through systematic questioning, definitional analysis, and precedent matching, enhancing consistency across reviewers and time periods.
- Contract and agreement analysis is one of the simplest AI applications in research administration, with natural language processing pulling out key terms, flagging risks, and verifying necessary provisions.
- Continuous compliance monitoring, tracking protocols, consent forms, adverse events, and regulatory submissions, shifts management from reactive to proactive.
- Conflict of interest management benefits from AI's capacity to systematically cross-reference financial disclosures with research activities and monitor compliance with management plans.

- Export control compliance now faces increased enforcement efforts; AI-supported screening helps institutions stay compliant with changing requirements at scale.
- Emerging research on LLMs for IRB review shows promise but raises important concerns about confidentiality, overreliance, and transparency.
- Governance frameworks from NIST and the Joint Commission/CHAI offer structure for institutions implementing AI in administrative roles.
- Ethical use requires ensuring efficiency gains don't compromise protections, auditing for algorithmic bias, and maintaining transparent, appealable decision processes.

QUESTIONS FOR REFLECTION

1. How can AI-supported research decisions enhance consistency at your institution while allowing appropriate flexibility for truly ambiguous cases?
2. Which compliance monitoring tasks take up the most administrator time at your institution, and which are most suitable for AI support?
3. How can you ensure AI administrative support improves rather than replaces human judgment on ethical issues?
4. What are the most important transparency measures when AI assists in administrative decisions that impact researchers?
5. How can AI assist your institution in more effectively managing multisite research compliance while honoring local context and requirements?
6. What confidentiality measures would you require before permitting AI systems to handle IRB applications that include sensitive research information?

NOTES

1. U.S. Department of Health and Human Services. (2017). Revised common rule. *Federal Register*, 82(12), 7149–7274. https://www.federalregister.gov/documents/2017/01/19/2017-01058/federal-

policy-for-the-protection-of-human-subjects. Note: Published January 19, 2017; compliance date January 21, 2019. The revised rule updated the definition of human subjects research, exemption categories, and single IRB requirements for multisite research.
2. U.S. Department of Health and Human Services. (2018). Exempt research determination FAQs. OHRP Guidance. https://www.hhs.gov/ohrp/regulations-and-policy/guidance/faq/exempt-research-determination/index.html. Note: The revised Common Rule significantly expanded exemption categories (45 CFR 46.104), adding new categories for benign behavioral interventions and secondary research with broad consent, while requiring limited IRB review for certain exempt categories involving identifiable information.
3. National Institute of Standards and Technology. (2023). Artificial intelligence risk management framework (AI RMF 1.0). NIST AI 100-1. https://www.nist.gov/itl/ai-risk-management-framework. Note: The framework's four core functions, Govern, Map, Measure, and Manage, provide applicable structure for institutions deploying AI in research administration, emphasizing accountability, risk-based oversight, and continuous monitoring.
4. The Joint Commission & Coalition for Health AI. (2025, September 17). The responsible use of AI in healthcare (RUAIH). https://www.jointcommission.org/en-us/knowledge-library/news/2025-09-jc-and-chai-release-initial-guidance-to-support-responsible-use-of-ai-in-health-care/. Note: This nonbinding guidance outlines seven actionable steps for healthcare organizations deploying AI, including governance structures, data protection, performance monitoring, bias mitigation, and workforce training. While developed for healthcare delivery, its governance framework is directly adaptable to research administration contexts.
5. U.S. Food and Drug Administration. (2023, August 15). Informed consent guidance for IRBs, clinical investigators, and sponsors. https://www.fda.gov/regulatory-information/search-fda-guidance-documents/informed-consent. Note: This final guidance, issued August 2023, supersedes earlier drafts and provides comprehensive recommendations for complying with informed consent requirements under 21 CFR Part 50. It addresses key information presentation, the consent process, documentation, and special situations including electronic consent methods.
6. U.S. Department of Commerce, Bureau of Industry and Security. (2024). Export administration regulations. 15 CFR 730-774. https://www.bis.doc.gov/index.php/regulations/export-administration-regulations-ear

7. U.S. Department of Commerce, Bureau of Industry and Security. (2024, August 14). Compliance note: Voluntary self-disclosure trends at academic research institutions. See also: Hogan Lovells. (2024, August 14). U.S. announces export enforcement and compliance resources for academic research institutions. https://www.hoganlovells.com/en/publications/us-announces-export-enforcement-and-compliance-resources-for-academic-research-institutions. Note: BIS highlighted common violations including unauthorized deemed exports to foreign national researchers, failure to classify controlled biological materials, and inadequate screening of international collaborators.
8. U.S. Department of Commerce, Bureau of Industry and Security. (2025, September 30). Interim final rule: 50 percent ownership threshold for Entity List and MEU List restrictions. See: Holland & Knight. (2025, October 5). BIS expands impact of U.S. export controls with 50 percent rule. https://www.hklaw.com/en/insights/publications/2025/10/bis-expands-impact-of-us-export-controls-with-50-percent-rule. Note: This rule automatically extends Entity List restrictions to companies 50% or more owned by listed entities, significantly expanding the scope of due diligence required for research partnerships involving commercial entities.
9. Mann, M., et al. (2025). Development of application-specific large language models to support IRB review processes. arXiv:2501.10741. https://arxiv.org/abs/2501.10741. Note: Proposes LLMs fine-tuned on IRB-specific documents and past review decisions for prereview screening, preliminary analysis, consistency checking, and decision support, with human-in-the-loop oversight.
10. Hosseini, M., et al. (2026). Guidelines needed for the use of AI in the preparation or review of research ethics applications. *BMC Medical Ethics*, 8, 2612564. https://pmc.ncbi.nlm.nih.gov/articles/PMC12823195/. Note: Highlights confidentiality risks when IRB applications containing sensitive participant information are submitted to AI tools, and the absence of clear contractual guarantees about data retention, usage, and sharing by AI system developers.
11. Public Responsibility in Medicine and Research (PRIM&R). (2025–2026). AI education programs for research oversight professionals. https://primr.org/programs/ai-education/. Note: PRIM&R has developed a comprehensive portfolio of AI-focused webinars, workshops, and symposia specifically for HRPP, IRB,

and IACUC professionals. Programs include hands-on AI training for administrative workflows (December 2025), a symposium on balancing AI innovation and research ethics (December 2025), webinars on IRB readiness for AI approvals (January 2026) and institutional AI innovations (April 2026), and an AI-driven behavioral analysis workshop for IACUC contexts (March 2026).

12. Public Responsibility in Medicine and Research (PRIM&R). (2025, January). Comments to NTIA on dual-use foundation models with widely available model weights. See: ITN Online. (2025, January 22). PRIM&R calls for 'clear and comprehensive guidance' on data used in AI. https://www.itnonline.com/content/primr-calls-clear-and-comprehensive-guidance-data-used-ai. Note: PRIM&R advocated for ethical guidelines governing research data used in AI development, emphasizing the need for clear frameworks addressing consent, privacy, and responsible data stewardship.

9 AI for IRB and Ethics Review Optimization

THE CHALLENGE OF IRB AND ETHICS REVIEW

Institutional review boards (IRBs) hold a unique role in the research world: they are responsible for protecting human research participants through strict ethical review, yet they must do so despite limited resources, increasing workloads, and growing complexity in the research they supervise. This tension between thoroughness and timeliness influences nearly every part of IRB functions.

The volume of reviews is substantial and growing. IRBs handle more protocols across diverse research areas, methodologies, and risk levels. Protocols have become more complex, often involving multisite collaborations, advanced technologies, and study designs that don't fit traditional review categories. The ratio of protocols to reviewers often requires quick reviews that may overlook important ethical considerations, a concerning issue when participant protection remains the main goal.

Consistency is perhaps the most persistent challenge to quality. Different reviewers examining similar protocols may reach different conclusions about risk levels, necessary protections, or the adequacy of consent. Some variation reflects genuine differences in ethical judgment, the kind of thoughtful diversity that makes multimember review valuable. However, when variation arises from different reviewers applying criteria inconsistently, or from some reviewers identifying issues that others overlook,

DOI 10.1201/9781003782995-12

inconsistency becomes a quality problem that weakens both protection and fairness.

Expertise gaps increase these challenges. Protocols are more often involving specialized methods (genomics, artificial intelligence [AI], and wearable biosensors), technologies (gene editing, brain–computer interfaces), or populations (indigenous communities, incarcerated persons, and individuals with cognitive impairments) that require knowledge not always found on any IRB. Securing enough expertise for each protocol, through board composition, consultants, or reviewer training, remains a continuous challenge for most institutions.

The regulatory landscape adds complexity. IRBs must follow the requirements of the Common Rule, applicable FDA regulations, HIPAA provisions for health information, and their own institutional policies, all while exercising ethical judgment that goes beyond simple regulatory compliance. The Belmont Report's principles of respect for persons, beneficence, and justice provide the ethical foundation, but turning these principles into specific decisions about individual protocols requires nuanced judgment that regulations alone cannot provide.[1]

AI has real potential to support IRB operations, not by replacing ethical debate, which remains fundamentally human work, but by managing routine tasks that consume reviewers' time and attention: checking completeness, verifying consistency, analyzing readability, retrieving precedents, and managing workload. By moving these routine analytical tasks to AI, IRBs can concentrate human effort where it truly counts, ethical reasoning and deliberative judgment that form the core of the board's work.

PROTOCOL REVIEW ASSISTANCE

AI can assist with multiple stages of protocol review while maintaining the importance of human ethical judgment. The most immediately useful applications are those that occur before human review begins, ensuring reviewers receive complete, consistent materials and relevant context.

PRELIMINARY ANALYSIS AND COMPLETENESS CHECKING

Before a protocol reaches a reviewer's desk, AI can perform systematic preliminary analysis: verifying that all required elements are included (research objectives, methods, participant selection, risk assessment, protection measures, consent processes, data management, and dissemination plans), checking internal consistency across protocol sections, identifying which specific regulatory requirements apply based on study characteristics, and flagging areas where protocols lack necessary information. This prescreening enables administrative staff to request clarifications before the protocol enters formal review, preventing the frustrating cycle of submission, incomplete review, return for additional information, and resubmission that wastes time for both reviewers and investigators.

Prior determination retrieval is one of AI's most valuable contributions to consistency. By identifying similar previously reviewed protocols and how they were assessed, including what determinations were made, what protections were required, and what concerns were raised, AI provides reviewers with a baseline that promotes consistent treatment of similar research. This doesn't mean that identical protocols must receive identical determinations (as circumstances, context, and knowledge evolve), but it ensures that reviewers are aware of relevant precedent when making new decisions.

RISK AND BENEFIT ASSESSMENT SUPPORT

Assessing whether research risks are reasonable in relation to anticipated benefits is the key ethical judgment in IRB review.[1] AI can support this judgment without replacing it. For risk identification, AI can systematically list potential physical, psychological, social, economic, and legal risks based on protocol features, helping ensure reviewers consider the full range of potential harms rather than just the most obvious ones. Estimating the risk magnitude, using published literature about similar interventions and procedures, provides an evidence-based context for assessing severity and likelihood. Additionally, identifying vulnerable populations, such as children, prisoners, pregnant women, cognitively impaired individuals, or economically disadvantaged persons, ensures that appropriate protection measures are triggered when necessary.

For benefit assessment, AI can help distinguish between benefits to direct participants, future patients or populations, and contributions to knowledge alone, a distinction that matters because the ethical considerations vary depending on the type of benefit expected. AI can also identify protocol language that might promote therapeutic misconception, participants' mistaken belief that research procedures are mainly designed for their personal benefit, a common problem in clinical research that well-crafted consent processes should address.

However, the final risk-benefit assessment, whether risks are justified by benefits, whether risks are properly minimized, and whether protections are adequate, requires the kind of value judgment and contextual reasoning that remains firmly within human decision-making authority.

CONSENT FORM ANALYSIS AND OPTIMIZATION

Informed consent is the practical expression of respecting individuals in research. AI can improve consent forms in measurable ways while helping achieve the larger goal of ensuring participants truly understand.

REQUIRED ELEMENTS AND REGULATORY COMPLIANCE

Federal regulations specify required elements for informed consent, purpose, procedures, duration, risks, benefits, alternatives, confidentiality protections, voluntary participation, right to withdraw, contact information, and provisions for compensation and injury.[2] Additional elements are necessary for specific populations (children, pregnant women, and prisoners) and regulatory contexts (FDA-regulated research, HIPAA-covered data). AI can systematically verify that consent forms include all applicable required elements by checking both federal requirements and institution-specific policies that might go beyond federal minimums. This comprehensive review helps identify gaps that human reviewers might overlook, especially when multiple regulatory frameworks are involved.

Consistency verification, ensuring consent forms accurately mirror the protocol regarding procedures, risks, benefits, and study design, is another area where AI truly adds value. Discrepancies between what a protocol describes and what a consent form informs participants of are both common and significant: they can mislead participants and lead to regulatory compliance issues. AI can systematically compare consent form descriptions against protocol text, flagging inconsistencies for review.

READABILITY AND COMPREHENSION

Perhaps the most well-documented issue with informed consent forms is their readability, or rather, their lack of it. The landmark study by Paasche-Orlow, Taylor, and Brancati found that templates for informed consent forms from U.S. medical schools averaged a 10.6 grade level on the Flesch-Kincaid scale, surpassing the IRBs' own recommended readability standards by an average of 2.8 grade levels.[3] Federal oversight was linked to improved readability, but even institutions with oversight still produced forms far above suggested reading levels. This issue, documented over 20 years ago, persists today: consent forms regularly contain dense medical and legal jargon, passive voice, and complex sentence structures that hinder many participants' understanding.

AI can address this systematically. Readability analysis using validated metrics (Flesch-Kincaid, SMOG, and Gunning Fog) provides an objective assessment of reading level requirements. More importantly, AI can identify specific passages that raise the reading level, overly complex sentences, technical jargon with available plain-language alternatives, unnecessarily long paragraphs, and suggest simplifications that preserve accuracy while enhancing accessibility. Structure assessment can evaluate whether consent forms use clear headings, logical flow, and proper organization to support comprehension rather than just ticking a regulatory box. Additionally, length evaluation can flag when consent forms have become so lengthy that they may overwhelm rather than inform participants, a particular challenge in multiarm clinical trials and genomic research.

Beyond basic readability, AI can enhance understanding by pinpointing the key information participants need for meaningful consent, as highlighted by the revised Common Rule's "key information" requirement. It can also predict questions participants might have based on the consent form, evaluate cultural relevance for targeted populations, and identify where visual aids, such as diagrams, flowcharts, or decision tools, might improve comprehension more effectively than additional text.

LITERATURE REVIEW AND PRECEDENT ANALYSIS

IRB review benefits from understanding existing evidence about research procedures, risks, and protections, context that individual reviewers may not have time to research for every protocol they review.

AI can effectively locate and synthesize published evidence relevant to evaluating research risks and benefits: identifying adverse event reports for proposed interventions, summarizing evidence about risk levels for specific procedures, finding published studies using similar methods with comparable populations, and monitoring whether the evidence base for a particular approach has changed since the protocol was created. This evidence synthesis does not replace reviewers' judgment in weighing evidence, but it ensures that judgments are informed by the best available data rather than relying solely on individual reviewers' knowledge.

Precedent analysis goes beyond an institution's previous decisions to tracking changing standards within the research ethics community. AI can monitor new guidance from OHRP, FDA, professional organizations, and international bodies, alert when protocols involve advanced methods needing updated ethical review, and detect when methodologies or populations are under ethical debate that reviewers should consider. The Secretary's Advisory Committee on Human Research Protections (SACHRP) has issued recommendations concerning AI-specific issues, including risks to nonsubjects impacted by AI research, group-level harms from algorithmic bias, and the need for frameworks to assess AI research ethically.[4] SACHRP's was disbanded in March 2025 after a review of all HHS discretionary committees.[5] Nonetheless, its existing recommendations provide essential guidance that AI systems can assist IRBs in systematically applying.

MEETING PREPARATION AND DOCUMENTATION

IRB meetings require thorough preparation and the creation of key documentation, with tasks where AI's efficiency can save staff time for more valuable work.

For premeeting preparation, AI can help organize agendas by grouping related protocols and efficiently arranging discussions. It can ensure that reviewers receive complete materials in clear, structured formats, identify protocols that may benefit from specific reviewer expertise or external advice, estimate discussion time based on complexity and past review patterns, and flag protocols likely to require extensive deliberation. These organizational tasks often require significant staff time and are better managed through systematic methods rather than ad hoc approaches.

Meeting documentation is particularly well-suited for AI support. IRBs need to keep detailed records of discussions, decisions, votes, and rationales, which are essential for accountability, regulatory compliance, and institutional memory. AI can generate draft minutes from meeting discussions for staff review, track follow-up action items, produce draft determination letters documenting decisions and necessary changes, and accurately record votes and conflicts of interest recusals. Postmeeting follow-up, such as monitoring correspondence with investigators, assessing whether responses sufficiently address IRB concerns, and generating final approval documentation, also benefits from systematic AI tracking to prevent anything from being overlooked.

WORKLOAD MANAGEMENT AND REVIEW EFFICIENCY

IRBs need to manage workloads effectively to provide prompt reviews without sacrificing quality, a balance that becomes harder to maintain as submission numbers increase.

REVIEW PATHWAY DETERMINATION

AI can assist in routing decisions that determine how efficiently protocols move through the system. Exemption screening identifies protocols that could qualify for exempt status, guiding them to the appropriate faster pathway. Expedited review identification recognizes protocols eligible for single-reviewer review instead of full board review. Continuing review frequency assessment aligns review schedules with risk profiles, ensuring high-risk studies get frequent oversight while lower-risk studies are not subjected to unnecessarily burdensome review cycles. Modification severity assessment determines whether protocol changes require full board review or expedited or administrative review, a triage decision that significantly affects both turnaround time and reviewer workload.

GOVERNANCE ALIGNMENT

IRBs implementing AI support tools should ensure these tools meet the same governance standards the IRB expects from AI research it reviews. This is a reflexive obligation that is both principled and practical. The NIST AI Risk Management Framework offers a structured approach through its Govern, Map, Measure, and Manage functions that IRBs can use to evaluate and oversee AI tools in their review processes.[6] The FUTURE-AI guideline, developed through international consensus among 117 experts from 50 countries, provides principles particularly relevant to IRB AI tools: traceability (ensuring AI analyses can be traced to their inputs and logic), usability (ensuring tools are practical for reviewers with varying technical skills), and explainability (ensuring AI outputs are interpretable rather than opaque).[7]

If an IRB cannot explain how its own AI tools produce their outputs, it is poorly positioned to demand explainability from the AI research it oversees.

REVIEWER ASSIGNMENT AND WORKLOAD DISTRIBUTION

Matching protocols to reviewers with suitable expertise is both important and logistically complex. AI can analyze reviewers' backgrounds, publications, and review histories to identify their areas of expertise and then match protocols to reviewers with relevant knowledge, ensuring that a protocol involving gene therapy, for instance, is assigned to someone with molecular biology expertise rather than simply based on workload. At the same time, AI can spot learning opportunities where junior reviewers can gain experience on appropriate protocols with proper senior oversight, help ensure review teams include diverse perspectives, distribute workload fairly across the reviewer pool, and detect conflicts of interest that require recusal, automating the process of finding suitable replacement reviewers when conflicts occur.

Reviewing timeline management, tracking how long protocols stay at each stage, highlighting unusual delays, monitoring regulatory deadlines, and generating performance metrics, provides the operational intelligence IRBs need to spot and fix bottlenecks before they cause backlogs.

QUALITY ASSURANCE AND IMPROVEMENT

Maintaining consistent, high-quality reviews across many protocols and reviewers requires systematic quality assurance, an area where AI's ability to analyze patterns in large numbers of reviews offers unique value.

REVIEW QUALITY AND INTERRATER RELIABILITY

AI can evaluate review quality by checking if reviews address all key considerations, spotting variation in how similar protocols are treated, recognizing when reviews could benefit from a deeper focus on specific issues, and highlighting especially thorough or insightful reviews that can help train reviewers. Interrater reliability analysis, which measures agreement between reviewers on important decisions and identifies reasons for disagreement, serves as the basis for calibration discussions that boost consistency without overly standardizing judgment.

Continuous improvement relies on aggregate data to enhance IRB processes over time: monitoring performance metrics (review times, approval rates, and modification request rates), detecting trends that suggest process enhancements or emerging issues, recognizing areas where reviewer training could fill knowledge gaps, and pinpointing workflow inefficiencies suitable for improvement. While these data-driven insights are difficult to produce manually, they are straightforward for AI systems with access to IRB records.

SPECIALIZED REVIEW SUPPORT

Certain protocols require specialized ethical consideration, which AI can help ensure is appropriately triggered and addressed.

VULNERABLE POPULATIONS

Research involving vulnerable populations requires enhanced protections, with specific requirements varying by group. AI can systematically identify when protocols involve populations needing special consideration, such as children, prisoners, pregnant women, cognitively impaired individuals, and economically disadvantaged persons, and verify that protocols include appropriate additional safeguards. For research involving children, AI can check whether studies provide the prospect of direct benefit as required by specific regulations, meet alternative criteria, and assess whether assent procedures are suitable for the developmental level of the proposed participants. For cognitively impaired adults, AI can evaluate whether consent processes incorporate suitable capacity assessments and surrogate decision-making provisions.

INTERNATIONAL AND CROSS-CULTURAL RESEARCH

Research conducted internationally or involving culturally diverse populations requires sensitivity to local norms, values, and power dynamics. AI can flag when protocols involve populations with specific cultural considerations, assess whether research approaches respect local norms, evaluate community engagement and consultation processes, and consider whether the benefit-risk balance is appropriate given the local context and available alternatives. However, genuine cultural competence, understanding how cultural dynamics affect research relationships and participant experiences, requires human knowledge, often including direct community engagement, that AI cannot provide.

EMERGING TECHNOLOGY RESEARCH

Research involving new technologies, gene editing, AI systems, brain–computer interfaces, and wearable biosensors presents ethical challenges that may not be fully addressed by current review frameworks. The MRCT Center and WCG released a Framework for Review of Clinical Research Involving AI in June 2025, providing IRBs with structured guidance for evaluating protocols where AI is part of the research intervention.[8] The framework features a decision tree for regulatory applicability, development-stage-specific review guidance, and targeted ethical considerations focusing on algorithmic bias, adaptive learning, data identifiability, and human oversight. Recently, Eto and colleagues introduced a Three-Stage Framework that matches IRB oversight intensity with an AI project's stage of maturity, from initial data-training phases (where risks concern data integrity and consent), through testing stages (where bias and safety issues arise), to deployment phases (where population-level impacts must be assessed).[9]

These frameworks show a growing recognition that review methods for AI need to be tailored to AI's unique traits: its iterative development, its potential for group-level rather than individual-level harm, and its ability to change after deployment in ways that may alter its risk profile.

EMERGING AI TOOLS FOR IRB OPERATIONS

The use of AI in IRB operations is transitioning from concept to practice. Mann and colleagues suggested developing application-specific large language models (LLMs) fine-tuned on IRB-related literature and institutional datasets, "Chat-IRB" systems capable of prereview screening, initial analysis, consistency checks, and decision support while keeping human oversight for all critical judgments.[10] Their proposal stresses that such systems should improve efficiency and quality while maintaining the IRB's core function of deliberative judgment, enhancing reviewers rather than replacing them.

However, deploying AI in IRB operations raises unique concerns. Hosseini and colleagues pointed out that submitting IRB applications to AI tools introduces confidentiality risks, especially when applications include sensitive participant data, unpublished research ideas, or proprietary methods.[11] Without explicit contractual assurances about data retention and usage, institutions cannot guarantee that uploaded content won't be stored by AI developers, used to train future models, or accessed by unauthorized individuals. They also expressed concern that AI could worsen existing tendencies toward checklist-driven, mechanistic reviews by further disconnecting reviewers from the ethical reasoning behind their decisions, a "deskilling" risk that institutions must actively prevent.

Commercial platforms are beginning to emerge. AI-powered protocol submission systems that guide investigators through structured questions, identify inconsistencies, detect missing elements, and verify regulatory compliance before protocols reach the IRB are already in use at some institutions. These systems shift some quality control tasks from reviewers to the submission phase, where making corrections is less costly for everyone involved. The AAHRPP hosted a webinar series in 2025 examining AI applications throughout the review process, from presubmission screening to postapproval monitoring, with a special focus on governance structures that ensure AI supports rather than replaces ethical deliberation.[12]

Similarly, PRIM&R has created targeted programs exploring these questions from various perspectives: their January 2026 webinar "AI and the IRB: When Are We Ready to Push 'Approved'?" addressed data privacy, transparency, and bias issues that IRBs need to consider before incorporating AI into approval processes, while their April 2026 session "AI in Action: Institutional Innovations Supporting IRB Review" highlights how institutions are developing practical methods for AI-supported review.[13]

PRACTICAL IMPLEMENTATION STRATEGIES

Implementing AI support for IRB operations requires maintaining the board's independence and careful decision-making process while achieving efficiency improvements.

MAINTAINING IRB AUTONOMY AND JUDGMENT

The core principle is that final decisions rest with IRB members, not algorithms. AI analyses should serve as starting points for discussion, not final answers, they should inform debate rather than limit it. AI systems must be able to explain their analyses so reviewers can understand the reasoning and evaluate it critically. Override options must be simple to use, and overrides should be common rather than rare, reflecting that ethical judgment often involves factors that systematic analysis cannot capture. Transparency about AI's role in review processes is crucial for maintaining trust among researchers and participants, though it doesn't need to include details of deliberative discussions.

TRAINING AND QUALITY CONTROL

Effective implementation requires training at multiple levels. IRB members need to understand what AI tools do, what they don't do, and when to trust or question their outputs. Staff need operational competence with AI systems and the ability to troubleshoot problems. Calibration exercises that use AI-supported analyses in training contexts to reveal and discuss reviewer variation can improve consistency while building reviewers' confidence in working with AI tools.

Validation is an ongoing process, not a one-time task. Accuracy checks, bias audits, performance assessments, and human reviews of AI outputs must be continuous, with findings feeding back into system improvements. If an AI tool repeatedly flags a protocol as high-risk while experienced reviewers view it as low-risk, the tool needs recalibration, and the pattern itself offers valuable insights into potential misalignments between the tool's training data or logic and current practices.

CAPABILITIES AND LIMITATIONS: THE IRB AND ETHICS AUDIT

While the Master Matrix in Chapter 1 outlines general AI strengths in Oversight Tasks and Regulatory Mapping, applying these to the IRB requires this book's most stringent Override Protocols. IRB review is not a checklist; it is an exercise in moral philosophy and community protection. AI can optimize the *workflow* of an IRB, but it cannot perform the *deliberation* that is the board's legal and ethical core (Table 9.1).

TABLE 9.1
IRB-Specific Override Protocols

IRB Task	AI Execution (The "Meat")	The Human Override (The Top Bread)
Risk evidence synthesis	Rapidly locating and integrating published data to assist in the Risk/Benefit analysis	**Clinical Sanity Check:** Humans must judge if the "evidence" is applicable to the specific local population. AI cannot weigh "incommensurable goods"
Consistency checking	Comparing protocols, consent forms, and prior board decisions to identify discrepancies	**Contextual Adaptation:** AI flags *deviations*; humans must determine if a deviation is a *justified* clinical necessity or an ethical lapse

(*Continued*)

TABLE 9.1 (*Continued*)
IRB-Specific Override Protocols

IRB Task	AI Execution (The "Meat")	The Human Override (The Top Bread)
Workload optimization	Matching protocols to reviewers based on expertise and balancing board assignments	**Conflict of Interest Audit:** AI maps *affiliations*; humans must sense *relationships*. Manually vet for subtle biases or professional rivalries the AI cannot "see"
Vulnerability screening	Scanning protocols for keywords related to protected or vulnerable populations	**Lived-Experience Assessment:** AI identifies "categories" of vulnerability; humans must understand the social circumstances that create actual risk

Refer to the Master Matrix in Chapter 1 for foundational failure modes; the table outlines the expert-level interventions required for ethical oversight.

THE MORAL REASONING GAP

A fundamental limitation of AI in the IRB context is its inability to engage in Ethical Deliberation. AI can simulate the *language* of ethics (e.g., quoting the Belmont Report), but it cannot perform the *act* of moral judgment.

- **The AI Limit**: AI cannot "weigh" competing values. It can tell you that a study has a 5% risk of a side effect, but it cannot decide if that risk is "respectful" of a participant's autonomy.
- **The Human Task**: You must provide the Value Judgment. The board must use AI-generated summaries as *input*, but the final "Approval" or "Disapproval" must result from human-to-human debate and the weighing of the Three Principles (Respect, Beneficence, and Justice).

COMMUNITY VALUES AND PROPORTIONALITY

IRB review relies on local knowledge and cultural competence that remain invisible to algorithms:

1. **Community Norms**: What is considered "acceptable risk" or "appropriate compensation" varies wildly between a rural clinic and an urban academic center. AI lacks the cultural competence to navigate these local sensitivities.
2. **The "Hidden" Vulnerability**: AI tracks formal categories (e.g., prisoners, children). It often misses "situational" vulnerability, such as a population with low digital literacy being asked to use a complex AI-driven health app.
3. **Proportionality versus Math**: AI can calculate if a payment is "statistically significant" compared to local wages. Only a human can judge if that payment constitutes undue inducement, a moral distinction, not a mathematical one.

The Override Trigger: If the AI suggests that a protocol is "Low Risk" based purely on keyword matching, but your professional intuition senses a threat to participant autonomy or community trust, you must trigger a Full Board Review Bypass. The IRB's mission is to protect humans; the AI's mission is to process data. When they conflict, the human must always override.

THE SKEPTIC'S CORNER

- **Target Task**: Protocol review and risk/benefit assessment.
- **Adversarial Prompt**: "I have drafted a response to the IRB's concerns about patient privacy. Identify any 'AI-speak' or technical jargon in my response that obfuscates the actual risk of re-identification, and rewrite it for a community board member."

ETHICAL CONSIDERATIONS

Using AI to support ethics review raises its own ethical questions, a recursive challenge that IRBs are uniquely positioned to understand.

PRESERVING DELIBERATIVE CHARACTER

IRB review is inherently deliberative. The exchange of perspectives, weighing of conflicting values, and integration of different viewpoints are not inefficiencies to be eliminated but the mechanisms through which ethical oversight maintains its quality. AI must not replace this deliberation with automated outputs, restrict discussion by presenting decisions as final, or homogenize judgment by pushing reviewers toward algorithmic consensus. Diversity of perspective is important in ethics review; AI that encourages too much uniformity would reduce review quality even if it appears to enhance efficiency.

ALGORITHMIC BIAS AND INNOVATION RISK

AI trained on historical review patterns may reproduce biases, systematically treating certain types of research, populations, or investigators differently than warranted. New research might be flagged as problematic just because it differs from the patterns in training data, creating an unintended innovation penalty. These biases need active monitoring and correction, acknowledging that the training data reflects human decisions that were themselves imperfect.

TRANSPARENCY, ACCOUNTABILITY, AND TRUST

IRBs must clearly define how AI supports their processes, both to preserve researcher trust and to ensure institutional accountability. Determination rationales should be accessible to investigators, appeal procedures must remain strong regardless of AI involvement in initial decisions, and transparent audit trails should record the basis for all decisions. Most importantly, IRBs must stay fully responsible for review decisions: AI involvement does not transfer or dilute accountability. When mistakes happen, and they will, there must be clear protocols for identifying, correcting, and learning from errors.

LOOKING FORWARD

AI capabilities for supporting IRB review continue to advance. Natural language understanding will enhance AI's ability to interpret protocol descriptions and identify ethical issues without needing structured input formats. Adaptive learning systems will improve through feedback while still maintaining human oversight, becoming better at spotting problems and suggesting relevant precedents as they review more protocols. Deliberation support tools might develop to assist (not replace) board discussions, perhaps by highlighting relevant considerations reviewers haven't yet mentioned or by offering structured frameworks for complex ethical analyses.

The regulatory landscape is also changing. Frameworks like the MRCT Center/WCG guidance and the Three-Stage Framework are starting to create structured methods for reviewing AI research, which will likely be improved as more experience is gained.[8,9] Institutions are developing AI-specific supplemental forms to prompt investigators to address AI-specific risks, bias, hallucinations, data privacy, and participant notification about AI involvement, ensuring IRBs get the information they need for informed review. Additionally, the growing body of research on AI in oversight is providing evidence-based recommendations to enhance both AI tools and the human processes they support.

However, the fundamental nature of IRB review, ethical deliberation about whether research adequately protects participants and aligns with the principles of respect for persons, beneficence, and justice, will remain primarily human work. The most promising path is AI that makes human deliberation more efficient, better informed, and more consistent, while humans retain full authority over the ethical judgments that define the IRB's mission.

CONCLUSION

IRBs bear a significant responsibility for protecting research participants and ensuring ethical research conduct. AI provides valuable support across all IRB functions: protocol analysis, risk assessment, consent form review, literature synthesis, meeting documentation, workload management, reviewer assignment, quality assurance, and specialized review support. These capabilities can improve review consistency, efficiency, and thoroughness, leading to better protection for participants and faster turnaround times for investigators.

But these capabilities should support rather than replace the ethical deliberation at the core of IRB review. AI manages systematic checking and information synthesis; IRB members provide ethical reasoning, contextual judgment, and moral deliberation. The aim is not to automate ethics but to free ethical reviewers to focus on the tasks only humans can perform and to ensure they have the evidence, context, and analytical support needed to do it effectively.

The next chapter examines how AI can assist a vital and quickly changing ethical review process: evaluating AI products themselves when they serve as research tools or interventions.

KEY TAKEAWAYS

- IRBs face increasing numbers of complex protocols with limited resources, causing tension between thorough review and speed that AI can help ease.
- AI assists with protocol review by performing initial completeness checks, verifying consistency, identifying risks, and retrieving prior determinations, handling systematic tasks so reviewers can focus on ethical judgment.
- Consent form analysis benefits from AI's ability to verify required elements, evaluate readability (a well-documented ongoing issue), check protocol-consent consistency, and recommend comprehension enhancements.
- Literature and precedent analysis ensure reviewer judgments are based on current evidence and align with institutional precedent.

- Multiple governance frameworks, including NIST AI RMF, FUTURE-AI, and the MRCT Center/WCG framework, provide structure for IRBs implementing AI tools and reviewing AI research.
- Emerging LLM-based approaches to IRB support show promise but raise confidentiality concerns and deskilling risks that require careful safeguards.
- Quality assurance through interrater reliability analysis and ongoing process monitoring ensures consistent, high-quality reviews.
- Ethical deliberation, moral reasoning, cultural competence, and proportionality judgment must remain the responsibilities of human IRB members; AI cannot replace these essential functions.
- IRBs deploying AI tools should adhere to the same governance standards they expect from the AI research they review.

QUESTIONS FOR REFLECTION

1. How might AI support enhance consistency in IRB review at your institution while maintaining the valuable diversity of perspectives that deliberation offers?
2. What aspects of protocol review take up the most reviewer time at your institution, and which are most suitable for AI support without compromising ethical oversight?
3. How can your IRB ensure that AI tools improve deliberation rather than promote a checklist-driven, mechanistic review?
4. What confidentiality measures would you need before permitting AI systems to handle IRB applications with sensitive research data?
5. How can AI-powered readability analysis support your institution in closing the ongoing gap between consent form reading levels and participant understanding?
6. If your IRB employs AI tools, should it disclose this to investigators and participants, and if so, how?

NOTES

1. National Commission for the Protection of Human Subjects of Biomedical and Behavioral Research. (1979). *The Belmont Report: Ethical Principles and Guidelines for the Protection of Human Subjects of Research*. U.S. Department of Health and Human Services. https://www.hhs.gov/ohrp/regulations-and-policy/belmont-report/index.html
2. U.S. Department of Health and Human Services. (2018). Informed consent requirements. 45 CFR 46.116. https://www.ecfr.gov/current/title-45/subtitle-A/subchapter-A/part-46
3. Paasche-Orlow, M. K., Taylor, H. A., & Brancati, F. L. (2003). Readability standards for informed-consent forms as compared with actual readability. *New England Journal of Medicine*, 348(8), 721–726. https://doi.org/10.1056/NEJMsa021212. Note: This cross-sectional study of 114 U.S. medical school IRBs found that consent form templates averaged a 10.6 grade level on the Flesch-Kincaid scale, exceeding IRBs' own stated readability standards by 2.8 grade levels. Federal oversight was associated with better (but still excessive) readability.
4. Secretary's Advisory Committee on Human Research Protections. (2023). IRB considerations on the use of artificial intelligence in human subjects research. U.S. Department of Health and Human Services. https://www.hhs.gov/ohrp/sachrp-committee/recommendations/irb-considerations-use-artificial-intelligence-human-subjects-research/index.html Note: SACHRP's recommendations address AI-specific concerns, including risks to non-subjects affected by AI research outcomes, group-level harms from algorithmic bias, considerations of justice when AI research disproportionately burdens certain communities, and the need for frameworks to evaluate AI research ethically.
5. https://www.hhs.gov/ohrp/sachrp-committee/index.html, accessed July 16, 2026. SACHRP was terminated as a discretionary committee on March 31, 2025.
6. National Institute of Standards and Technology. (2023). Artificial intelligence risk management framework (AI RMF 1.0). NIST AI 100-1. https://www.nist.gov/itl/ai-risk-management-framework
7. Lekadir, K., et al. (2025). FUTURE-AI: International consensus guideline for trustworthy and deployable artificial intelligence in healthcare. *BMJ*, 388, e081554. https://doi.org/10.1136/bmj-2024-081554. Erratum in: *BMJ*, 388, r340. https://doi.org/10.1136/bmj.r340. PMID: 39909534; PMCID: PMC11795397. Note: Developed through international consensus among 117

experts from 50 countries over 24 months using a modified Delphi approach, the FUTURE-AI framework comprises 30 recommendations organized around six guiding principles: Fairness, Universality, Traceability, Usability, Robustness, and Explainability.

8. Multi-Regional Clinical Trials Center of Brigham and Women's Hospital and Harvard & WCG. (2025, June 24). Framework for review of clinical research involving AI. https://mrctcenter.org/resource/framework-for-review-of-clinical-research-involving-ai/. Note: Developed through a multidisciplinary task force of IRB chairs, ethicists, AI technologists, and industry representatives, this framework provides a decision tree for regulatory applicability, development-stage-specific review guidance, and ethical considerations addressing algorithmic bias, adaptive learning, data identifiability, and human oversight in AI research.
9. Eto, T., Miller, H., Vidal, D., & Lifson, M. (2026). Streamlining IRB review of AI human subjects research (AIHSR): The three-stage framework. *Frontiers in Systems Biology*, 6, 1804193. https://doi.org/10.3389/fsysb.2026.1804193. Note: Proposes a risk-based oversight model aligning IRB review intensity with an AI project's development stage: Stage 1 (data training: focus on data integrity, consent, and scientific rigor), Stage 2 (testing: focus on bias, safety, and performance), and Stage 3 (deployment: focus on population-level impacts and ongoing monitoring).
10. Mann, S. P., Seah, J. J., Latham, S., Savulescu, J., Aboy, M., & Earp, B. D. (2025). Chat-IRB? How application-specific language models can enhance research ethics review. *Journal of Medical Ethics*, 14, 2025–110845. https://doi.org/10.1136/jme-2025-110845. Note: Proposes LLMs fine-tuned on IRB-specific literature, institutional policies, and past review decisions for prereview screening, preliminary analysis, consistency checking, and decision support, with mandatory human oversight for all substantive determinations.
11. Hosseini, M., Eisenman, D., Riddle, J., Pyle, S., Peters, A., Cobb, N., & Holmes, K. (08 Jan 2026): Guidelines needed for the use of AI in the preparation or review of IRB, IBC, and IACUC applications, Accountability in Research, https://doi.org/10.1080/08989621.2025.2612564. Note: Highlights confidentiality risks when applications containing sensitive participant information, unpublished ideas, or proprietary methods are submitted to AI tools and argues that AI could worsen checklist-driven,

mechanistic review by further disconnecting reviewers from ethical reasoning. Calls for urgent guidance and maintains that humans must always be the final decision-makers in research ethics oversight.

12. Association for the Accreditation of Human Research Protection Programs. (2025, October 1). HRPP innovations webinar: Should we use AI to support the IRB review process? It depends (of course!). https://www.aahrpp.org/docs/default-source/past-webinars/october-2025-hrpp-innovations-final.pdf?sfvrsn=d3d82a6e_1. Note: Explored AI use cases across the review lifecycle, from presubmission quality checks through postapproval monitoring, with emphasis on governance structures, human-in-the-loop oversight requirements, and matching AI capabilities to appropriate review stages.
13. Public Responsibility in Medicine and Research (PRIM&R). (2025–2026). AI education programs for research oversight professionals. https://primr.org/programs/ai-education/. Note: PRIM&R's AI-focused programming includes webinars specifically addressing AI in IRB operations: "AI and the IRB: When Are We Ready to Push 'Approved'?" (January 2026) explored data privacy, transparency, and bias in AI-supported approval workflows, and "AI in Action: Institutional Innovations Supporting IRB Review" (April 2026) examines institutional approaches to AI-supported review.

10 IRB and IACUC Review of AI Products in Research

THE CHALLENGE OF REVIEWING AI IN RESEARCH

When artificial intelligence (AI) is the research tool or intervention under study, rather than merely supporting administrative functions, institutional review boards (IRBs) and IACUCs confront a category of review challenge fundamentally different from traditional protocol assessment. The distinctive properties of AI systems create risks and ethical considerations that existing frameworks address imperfectly.

The most immediate challenge is opacity. Many powerful AI systems, particularly deep learning models, function as "black boxes" where the reasoning behind specific outputs resists straightforward explanation. A neural network with millions of parameters identifying complex, nonlinear patterns may produce accurate predictions without providing reasoning that humans can understand, or that IRB members can evaluate for safety and appropriateness. This opacity complicates every dimension of ethical review: risk assessment becomes harder when the mechanism of action is opaque, informed consent becomes harder when neither investigators nor participants can fully explain what the AI does, and accountability becomes diffuse when no one can articulate why a particular output was produced.

Dynamic behavior compounds the opacity problem. Unlike traditional interventions with fixed characteristics, a drug has a defined chemical composition, a surgical procedure follows a specified

DOI 10.1201/9781003782995-13

technique, and AI systems may adapt and change behavior based on the data they encounter, potentially developing properties during a study that weren't present at its outset.[1] This adaptability is often precisely what makes AI valuable, but it means that the system an IRB approves at protocol submission may differ meaningfully from the system operating 6 months into the study.

Bias and fairness concerns are pervasive. AI systems can perpetuate or amplify biases present in training data, potentially leading to discriminatory outcomes that differentially affect certain populations. Obermeyer and colleagues' landmark study demonstrated this concretely: a widely used algorithm for identifying patients needing extra care exhibited significant racial bias, reducing the number of Black patients identified for additional support by more than half, not through explicit racial criteria but because the algorithm used healthcare costs as a proxy for health needs, and Black patients historically generated lower costs at equivalent levels of illness.[2] This example illustrates how bias can enter through seemingly neutral design choices, making it invisible without deliberate fairness evaluation.

AI also introduces risk categories that don't fit traditional frameworks: algorithmic discrimination affecting populations beyond direct research participants, privacy breaches through AI-enabled reidentification of supposedly deidentified data, automation bias where clinicians or researchers overrely on AI recommendations and stop exercising independent judgment, and emergent harms from unexpected system behaviors that couldn't have been anticipated from understanding the system's individual components.

Regulatory uncertainty adds practical complexity. Determining whether an AI system is a medical device requiring FDA oversight, software as a medical device (SaMD), clinical decision support (CDS) software exempt from device regulation, or simply a research tool requiring only IRB review involves navigating classifications that are themselves evolving.[3] And the pace of AI innovation means that ethical frameworks and review processes struggle to keep current with technological capabilities, a gap that governance frameworks are only beginning to close.

Finally, expertise gaps present a structural challenge. Reviewing AI-enabled research requires understanding algorithmic approaches, training methodologies, validation strategies, and potential failure modes, technical knowledge that many IRB and IACUC members lack. Even when integration challenges can be anticipated, workflow disruptions, user resistance, and automation complacency, the specific risks depend on contextual factors that require both technical and domain expertise to evaluate.

These challenges don't render traditional ethical principles irrelevant. Beneficence, justice, and respect for persons remain the foundation of ethical review. But their application to AI-enabled research demands new frameworks, new expertise, and heightened attention to issues that traditional review processes weren't designed to address.

HEALTHCARE AI GOVERNANCE FRAMEWORKS

Building on the governance principles introduced in Chapter 9, three complementary governance frameworks have emerged, providing IRBs with structured approaches to evaluating AI in research. Understanding their distinct contributions and how they work together is essential for effective review.

JOINT COMMISSION/COALITION FOR HEALTH AI (CHAI) RUAIH FRAMEWORK

The Joint Commission and CHAI released the Responsible Use of AI in Healthcare (RUAIH) framework in September 2025, establishing seven elements for healthcare organizations deploying AI: formal governance structures with designated AI leadership and risk-based oversight; patient privacy and transparency policies; data security and data use protections including encryption, access controls, and security assessments; ongoing quality monitoring through risk-based validation and performance evaluation; voluntary, blinded reporting of AI safety-related events to enable cross-institutional learning; risk and bias assessment processes to identify, evaluate, and mitigate biases; and education and training for all AI users.[4]

While RUAIH was designed for clinical AI deployment rather than research, its principles translate directly to IRB review. Research institutions should have governance structures aligned with RUAIH principles. RUAIH's emphasis on ongoing quality monitoring informs what IRBs should require for AI performance surveillance during studies. Its bias assessment framework models what IRBs should expect from protocols involving AI. Its training standards suggest what researchers and staff need when conducting AI research. And its voluntary reporting framework could extend to research contexts, enabling cross-institutional learning from AI-related adverse events.

FUTURE-AI INTERNATIONAL CONSENSUS GUIDELINE

The FUTURE-AI framework, developed through international consensus among 117 interdisciplinary experts from 50 countries, provides approximately 30 best practices organized around six principles: Fairness (ensuring AI systems perform equitably across diverse populations), Universality (ensuring broad applicability across settings and contexts), Traceability (maintaining comprehensive documentation throughout the AI lifecycle), Usability (ensuring practical integration into workflows), Robustness (building systems that perform reliably under varying conditions), and Explainability (providing understandable explanations appropriate to user needs).[5]

For research contexts, FUTURE-AI's principles inform what IRBs should expect from AI systems used in or studied through research protocols. Its emphasis on traceability, comprehensive documentation of data sources, model architecture, training procedures, and validation approaches, provides a standard for protocol documentation requirements. Its attention to fairness across populations informs bias evaluation expectations. And its robustness principles guide assessment of whether AI systems are sufficiently reliable for research deployment.

NIST AI RISK MANAGEMENT FRAMEWORK

The NIST AI RMF provides a structured, sector-agnostic approach to managing AI risks through four core functions: Govern (establishing policies, accountability structures, and oversight mechanisms), Map (understanding AI system context, intended purposes, stakeholders, and potential impacts), Measure (assessing system characteristics and capabilities using appropriate metrics), and Manage (allocating resources to address identified risks through mitigation and monitoring).[6] The framework's emphasis on iterative application throughout the AI lifecycle, rather than one-time assessment, aligns well with IRB continuing review responsibilities.

INTEGRATING THE FRAMEWORKS

These frameworks are complementary rather than competing. NIST provides the risk management structure, FUTURE-AI provides lifecycle-specific best practices, and RUAIH translates both into healthcare operational requirements. IRBs can draw from all three: using NIST's Map function to understand AI system context and risks, FUTURE-AI principles to assess whether systems meet international best practices, RUAIH elements to verify healthcare-appropriate implementation plans, and NIST's Measure and Manage functions to ensure ongoing monitoring is adequate.

ALGORITHM TRANSPARENCY AND EXPLAINABILITY

Understanding how AI systems work is vital for ethical review, but many modern AI methods resist the kind of simple explanation that traditional approaches provide.

THE BLACK-BOX PROBLEM AND LEVELS OF TRANSPARENCY

The tension between AI capability and AI transparency is real and unlikely to be fully resolved. The most powerful AI models, large neural networks, transformer architectures, and deep learning systems, are often the least interpretable, while more interpretable approaches (decision trees, linear models, and rule-based systems) may sacrifice accuracy. IRBs must navigate this tradeoff rather than simply demanding full explainability, which may be neither achievable nor optimal.

What IRBs can reasonably require is transparency at multiple levels. Purpose transparency, understanding what the AI system is designed to do, is always achievable even when internal workings are opaque. Training data transparency, knowing what data trained the system, including demographic composition and potential biases, is essential for bias assessment. Performance transparency, understanding accuracy across contexts and populations, enables risk evaluation without requiring mechanistic understanding. Limitation transparency, clear documentation of known failure modes and populations for which the system performs poorly, enables informed risk-benefit analysis. And for consequential decisions affecting participants directly (diagnosis, treatment recommendations, and participant selection), some level of decision transparency about why specific outputs were produced should be expected.

Post hoc explainability methods, LIME, SHapley Additive exPlanations, and attention mechanisms, can provide explanations after model predictions, though IRBs should be aware that such explanations are approximations that may not faithfully represent the model's actual reasoning.[7] When possible and appropriate, inherently interpretable models may be preferable for research applications where understanding the mechanism matters, even at some cost to predictive accuracy.

DOCUMENTATION REQUIREMENTS

IRBs should require comprehensive AI system documentation aligned with emerging standards. This includes detailed model architecture descriptions, training methodology (data sources, preprocessing, augmentation, and validation approaches), comprehensive performance metrics across relevant populations, explicit documentation of known limitations and failure modes, clear version control (since updates may meaningfully change behavior), and ongoing monitoring plans for detecting performance degradation during research. Consider requiring Model Cards or similar standardized documentation, such as CHAI's Applied Model Card, that systematically capture AI tool characteristics, testing results, limitations, and bias assessments.[4]

BIAS, FAIRNESS, AND EQUITY ASSESSMENT

AI systems can perpetuate or amplify societal biases, creating ethical obligations that IRBs must take seriously. The Obermeyer study demonstrated how even well-intentioned algorithms can produce discriminatory outcomes through design choices that seem neutral on their face but reflect structural inequalities in the underlying data.[2]

SOURCES AND ASSESSMENT OF BIAS

Bias can enter AI systems at every stage: through training data that underrepresents certain populations or contains biased labels, through historical patterns reflecting past discrimination that algorithms learn and perpetuate, through measurement approaches that work differently across populations, through evaluation methods that assess only aggregate performance without examining subgroup differences, and through deployment in contexts or with populations different from those in development.[8]

Multiple definitions of fairness exist, demographic parity, equalized odds, predictive parity, individual fairness, counterfactual fairness, and achieving one form may preclude others. No single definition satisfies all intuitions about what fairness requires, and the appropriate definition depends on the research context and the consequences of different types of errors. IRBs should require researchers to choose and justify fairness metrics appropriate to their context, report disaggregated performance across relevant demographic groups, evaluate differential impacts, and acknowledge tradeoffs between competing fairness definitions.

Following RUAIH's guidance on bias assessment, IRBs should expect protocols to document training data representativeness, vendor or developer bias testing, population-appropriate validation (including local testing), and plans for ongoing bias monitoring.[4] Predeployment testing across populations, diverse validation datasets, and explicit documentation of residual biases that couldn't be fully mitigated should all be standard expectations.

Beyond technical mitigation, equity requires attention to who develops AI systems. Development teams should include diverse perspectives, affected communities should be consulted (not merely informed) about AI design and development, and cultural appropriateness should be evaluated for the populations the AI will affect. RUAIH specifically calls for governance structures that include "stakeholders reflecting the needs of impacted populations," a standard IRBs can apply to research contexts.[4]

SAFETY, VALIDATION, AND PERFORMANCE EVALUATION

IRBs must assess whether AI systems are sufficiently safe, validated, and reliable for research use, a determination that requires understanding both what validation means for AI and what ongoing monitoring research protocols must include.

VALIDATION STANDARDS

AI systems require multilayered validation before research deployment. Internal validation (performance on held-out development data) is necessary but insufficient, systems routinely perform better on data similar to their training data than on truly independent data. External validation on independent datasets from different sources establishes generalizability. For clinical AI, prospective validation in real-world conditions provides the strongest evidence of reliability. Subgroup validation, assessing performance across demographic and clinical subgroups, not just aggregate metrics, is essential for identifying disparate performance that aggregate statistics may mask. Temporal validation confirms that performance holds in current conditions when models were trained on historical data. And local validation, testing in the specific deployment context, even for FDA-authorized tools, addresses the reality that AI performance can vary significantly across institutional settings.[4]

ONGOING QUALITY MONITORING

Perhaps the most important adaptation for AI research protocols is the requirement for continuous performance monitoring during the study, not just predeployment validation and poststudy analysis. Protocols should specify how AI tools will be regularly tested for performance and reliability, how data quality will be evaluated (such as comparing AI outputs to known parameters), how use-case-relevant outcomes will be monitored, how adverse events potentially related to AI will be detected and reported, and what performance thresholds trigger revalidation, protocol modification, or study termination.

Drift detection deserves particular attention. Concept drift (when relationships between inputs and outputs change over time), data drift (when input distributions shift from training data), and performance degradation all threaten the validity and safety of AI research. Automated monitoring systems for detecting drift, clearly defined revalidation triggers, and stopping criteria for when degradation crosses safety thresholds should be standard protocol elements.

Understanding how AI systems fail is equally important. IRBs should assess known failure modes, whether systems fail safely or catastrophically, whether they can detect out-of-distribution inputs (data unlike their training data), what human oversight is required to catch and correct errors, and how errors are handled when they occur. RUAIH's emphasis on "keeping humans in the decision-making process" provides a useful touchstone: higher-risk applications demand closer human oversight, not less.[4]

RUAIH's emphasis on "keeping humans in the decision-making process" provides a useful touchstone: higher-risk applications demand closer human oversight, not less.[4] To operationalize this oversight, research protocols should define specific Override Criteria: predefined "Red Flags" that require a researcher to immediately bypass AI-generated results in favor of manual expert judgment. These criteria serve as the functional mechanism for countering automation bias and include:

- **Data Incongruity**: When AI outputs or summaries directly contradict verified primary data, established physiological realities, or the researcher's direct clinical observations.
- **Logical Black Boxes**: When an AI provides a conclusion or recommendation that lacks a transparent, traceable evidence chain, thereby violating the "Traceability" and "Explainability" requirements of the FUTURE-AI and NIST AI RMF frameworks.
- **Ethical Friction**: When an AI-generated suggestion conflicts with the core tenets of the Belmont Report: specifically the principles of Respect for Persons, Beneficence, and Justice, or with institutional clinical ethics guidelines.

By mandating these Override Triggers within the protocol, IRBs can ensure that human accountability is not merely a theoretical presence but a documented, active component of the research lifecycle. For a detailed discussion on the operationalization of these criteria via the "Sandwich Workflow," see Chapter 1.

INFORMED CONSENT FOR AI-ENABLED RESEARCH

Obtaining meaningful informed consent for research involving AI presents challenges that go beyond those of conventional interventions, precisely because AI's complexity, opacity, and adaptability make it harder for participants to understand what they're agreeing to.

DISCLOSURE AND COMPREHENSION

Consent forms for AI research should disclose that AI systems are involved, what roles they play, what the AI can and cannot do (including known limitations and error rates), whether and how AI decisions can be explained, whether the AI adapts during the study, what human oversight accompanies AI use, what alternatives exist, and how participant data may be used in AI training or broader development beyond the immediate study.

The comprehension challenge is substantial. AI concepts, machine learning, neural networks, and algorithmic decision-making, are unfamiliar to most participants. The decision-making processes are abstract and resist intuitive analogy. When novel AI approaches are involved, uncertainty about risks may be genuinely substantial rather than merely difficult to quantify. And participants may struggle to compare AI-related risks to familiar risks because the risk categories themselves are unfamiliar.

IRBs should assess whether consent materials make AI involvement genuinely comprehensible to intended participants, potentially requiring simplified explanations, analogies, visual aids, or layered consent approaches that provide key information prominently while making technical details available for those who want them. The revised Common Rule's emphasis on presenting "key information" first is particularly relevant for AI consent, where the volume of technical detail can overwhelm the essential information participants need for meaningful decision-making.

Specific consent considerations include explicit disclosure and consent for data use in algorithm training beyond the immediate study, explanation of reidentification risks (AI systems may enable reidentification of supposedly deidentified data), transparent acknowledgment that AI may perform differently for different populations, clarification of whether AI outputs are recommendations subject to human review or automated decisions with limited human involvement, whether participants can request human review of AI-mediated decisions, and how participants will be notified if AI systems change materially during the study. For vulnerable populations, participants with cognitive impairments, children, and individuals with limited English proficiency or health literacy, these comprehension challenges require especially careful attention and adapted consent approaches.

PRIVACY, DATA PROTECTION, AND SECURITY

AI systems typically process substantial personal data for training, operation, and validation, creating privacy obligations that extend beyond traditional research data protections.

DATA GOVERNANCE PRINCIPLES

IRBs should assess whether AI research protocols observe fundamental data governance principles: collecting only necessary data (data minimization), limiting use to specified purposes (purpose limitation), defining appropriate retention periods and disposition after research completion, obtaining explicit consent for secondary uses such as broader AI development, and establishing clear terms for any data sharing with other researchers, institutions, or AI developers.

When protected health information is involved, HIPAA compliance requires appropriate Business Associate Agreements with AI vendors, application of the minimum necessary standard, and safeguards commensurate with risk. Deidentification standards, Safe Harbor or Expert Determination, must be properly applied, though IRBs should be aware that even properly deidentified data may carry reidentification risks when processed by AI systems capable of pattern recognition and dataset linkage. Data use agreements should clearly define permitted uses, explicitly prohibit reidentification, require third-party vendor compliance with security standards, and reserve institutional audit rights.[4]

AI-SPECIFIC PRIVACY RISKS

AI creates privacy risks beyond those of conventional data handling. Pattern recognition may enable reidentification of deidentified data. Linkage attacks, combining datasets in ways that reveal identities, become more feasible with AI's ability to detect subtle correlations across large datasets. Inference attacks can derive sensitive attributes from nonsensitive data. And model inversion, where the AI model itself leaks information about its training data, represents a risk category unique to machine learning systems.[9]

Privacy-preserving techniques can mitigate some of these risks. Differential privacy provides mathematical guarantees about information leakage.[10] Federated learning enables multisite AI research without centralizing participant data. Synthetic data generation can reduce reliance on real participant data for some purposes. However, each technique involves privacy-utility tradeoffs that affect AI performance and research validity, tradeoffs that protocols should document and justify.

REGULATORY CLASSIFICATION AND OVERSIGHT

Determining appropriate regulatory oversight for AI in research involves classification questions that significantly affect study requirements, validation costs, and institutional timelines. As of early 2026, the landscape has shifted from localized FDA standards to a globally harmonized quality framework.

THE QUALITY MANAGEMENT SYSTEM REGULATION (QMSR) AND ISO 13485:2016 INTEGRATION

The most significant structural change in recent years occurred on February 2, 2026, when the FDA officially replaced the legacy Quality System Regulation with the Quality Management System Regulation (QMSR). This rule harmonized 21 CFR Part 820 with ISO 13485:2016,[11] the international standard for medical device quality management systems (QMSs).

For researchers and IRBs, this means that any AI system classified as a medical device must now be developed and maintained under a QMS that emphasizes risk-based internal audits and lifecycle traceability. AI tools operating under pre-2026 "check-the-box" validation protocols are now technically noncompliant with the unified FDA/ISO standard. This harmonization is particularly relevant for multisite international trials, as a single QMSR-compliant QMS now satisfies both U.S. and many international regulatory entry requirements.[12]

SAMD

The FDA continues to regulate software functions as medical devices based on their intended use. Risk classification (Class I, II, or III) remains dependent on the potential harm to the patient and the level of influence the AI has on a clinical decision.

The January 2025 FDA Final Guidance on AI-Enabled Device Software Functions codified the Total Product Life Cycle (TPLC) approach as the industry standard.[13] Submissions for AI-enabled research tools must now include comprehensive model descriptions, data lineage, and performance metrics tied specifically to clinical claims.

A cornerstone of this TPLC approach is the Predetermined Change Control Plan (PCCP). Following the 2025 guidance, PCCPs allow investigators to prespecify and obtain authorization for intended modifications to an adaptive AI system before they are implemented.[13] This is no longer an experimental pathway; it is the mandatory mechanism for research involving algorithms that learn or drift after deployment. With over 1,200 AI-enabled devices authorized by the FDA as of early 2026, these classification and TPLC requirements are now a foundational component of every clinical research protocol.[13]

CDS EXEMPTIONS

Some AI systems function as CDS tools with specific regulatory considerations. The FDA updated its CDS guidance in January 2026, superseding the 2022 version and clarifying the scope of software functions excluded from the medical device definition under the 21st Century Cures Act.[3] The updated guidance notably provides enforcement discretion for CDS software that produces only one clinically appropriate option (previously, such software would have failed the exclusion criteria), revises FDA's approach to time-critical CDS use, and adjusts recommendations regarding automation bias and independent review requirements.[3] IRBs should coordinate with regulatory experts when research involves potential SaMD or CDS to ensure appropriate classification, as misclassification can lead to either inadequate oversight or unnecessary regulatory burden.

INTERNATIONAL REGULATORY CONSIDERATIONS

AI research conducted internationally faces varying regulatory frameworks. The EU Medical Device Regulation and In Vitro Diagnostic Regulation apply European standards. The WHO has continued developing AI governance frameworks, with its March 2025 guidance on large multimodal models providing the most detailed operational guidance to date, assigning governments responsibility for setting performance baselines and requiring developers to supply documentation, enable independent audits, and maintain real-world monitoring.[13] The AIRIS 2025 conference, cohosted by WHO and Korea's MFDS, produced an outcome statement urging lifecycle, risk-proportionate governance across jurisdictions.[14] Multinational AI research requires coordination across these evolving frameworks, a practical challenge that IRBs should assess in protocol review.

CONTINUOUS LEARNING AND ADAPTIVE SYSTEMS

AI systems that learn and adapt during research deployment create oversight challenges that existing continuing review frameworks weren't designed to address. These adaptive systems may drift from validated performance as they learn from real-world data, learn inappropriate patterns from biased deployment data, produce emergent behaviors through adaptation, or amplify rather than correct errors through feedback loops.

IRBs should assess whether adaptive or locked algorithms are appropriate for a given study. Locked algorithms, fixed after initial training and validation, are simpler to oversee and provide stable risk profiles throughout a study. Adaptive algorithms offer potential performance improvements but introduce uncertainty about how the system will change. Hybrid approaches with periodic supervised retraining rather than continuous adaptation may balance these considerations. For higher-risk applications, locked algorithms are generally safer and more appropriate, a position consistent with RUAIH's risk-based oversight approach.[4]

When adaptive systems are used, enhanced oversight is essential: more frequent performance monitoring, clearly defined revalidation triggers, rollback capabilities to revert to previous versions if adaptation produces problems, comprehensive records of how systems change, and protocols for determining whether and how to notify participants that the AI system affecting them has materially changed.

ADVERSE EVENT REPORTING AND LEARNING SYSTEMS

AI-related adverse events, unsafe recommendations, performance degradation, biased outputs, integration failures, and automation bias incidents require reporting structures adapted to AI's distinctive characteristics.

Existing safety reporting systems (IRB adverse event reporting, institutional patient safety systems) can be leveraged rather than creating entirely new structures, but they need updating to capture AI-specific information: whether AI was involved, how it contributed, what the failure mode was, and whether the event reflects a systematic problem versus an isolated incident.[4] For FDA-regulated AI devices, existing adverse event reporting pathways apply. For nondevice AI, voluntary blinded reporting to independent organizations, as RUAIH envisions, enables cross-institutional learning without compromising patient privacy or institutional identity. Reporting through federally listed Patient Safety Organizations provides another protected pathway for confidential sharing.

The value of cross-institutional learning from AI adverse events cannot be overstated. Patterns that wouldn't be visible from single-site data, a particular AI system underperforming for a specific population, a failure mode that appears only under certain data conditions, become identifiable when events are aggregated across institutions. IRBs should require protocols to include plans for identifying, reporting internally, and sharing AI-related adverse events with the broader community through appropriate channels.

AI IN ANIMAL RESEARCH: IACUC CONSIDERATIONS

AI use in animal research creates specific IACUC considerations that extend beyond traditional protocol review. The ethical framework for animal research, built around the Three Rs principles of Replacement, Reduction, and Refinement, provides natural categories for evaluating AI's contribution.

THREE RS OPPORTUNITIES

AI offers genuine potential to advance each of the Three Rs. For replacement, predictive modeling of biological responses may reduce animals needed for preliminary testing, virtual screening of compounds may reduce testing of unpromising candidates, and cross-species translation models may improve the efficiency of translational research. For reduction, AI analysis of tissue samples and experimental data may extract more information from fewer animals, and optimized experimental designs informed by AI may achieve statistical power with smaller sample sizes. For refinement, AI-powered behavioral monitoring can detect pain or distress earlier than human observation, automated monitoring reduces handling stress while improving welfare oversight, and precision interventions guided by AI may be more accurate and less traumatic.

IACUCs should encourage AI approaches that meaningfully advance the Three Rs while maintaining scientific validity. However, several ethical considerations are specific to animal AI research. Using AI in treatment groups while withholding it from controls may create differential welfare outcomes requiring justification. AI systems must be adequately validated before deployment in animal research, poorly performing systems waste animal lives on unreliable results. Failure protocols must specify what happens to animals if AI systems malfunction during research. And the anticipated benefits of AI-enabled research must justify the animal use involved.

Hosseini and colleagues emphasized that IACUC review presents particular challenges for AI assistance because protocols require assessment of humane endpoints, species-specific enrichment adequacy, serial procedure implications, and the balance between scientific objectives and animal distress, judgments requiring veterinary expertise and contextual ethical reasoning that AI cannot currently provide.[15] AI cannot substitute for the deliberative, multidisciplinary assessment that the *Guide for the Care and Use of Laboratory Animals* requires, though it can support completeness checking and consistency verification in protocol review.

CAPABILITIES AND LIMITATIONS: THE AI-AS-SUBJECT AUDIT

While the Master Matrix in Chapter 1 outlines general AI strengths in Pattern Recognition and Regulatory Mapping, reviewing AI as a research intervention (the subject of the study) requires an entirely different set of Safety Override Triggers.

In previous chapters, I addressed AI as a tool for the researcher, in which failure modes include errors in documentation or synthesis. In this chapter, we shift to AI as the intervention under study. Here, the stakes escalate from administrative inaccuracy to Direct Participant Risk. If a study-investigational AI fails due to biased output, "black-box" logic, or performance drift, the result is not a faulty citation but potential clinical harm to the human or animal subject relying on that algorithm's output (Table 10.1).

TABLE 10.1
AI-Review Override Protocols

Review Category	AI Intervention Role (The Subject)	The Board-Mandated Override (The Top Bread)
Diagnostic/decision support	The AI under study provides a treatment trigger or diagnostic finding	**Clinical Confirmation**: The protocol must mandate that a human clinician confirms the AI's "finding" before any irreversible clinical action or treatment change is taken

(*Continued*)

TABLE 10.1 (*Continued*)
AI-Review Override Protocols

Review Category	AI Intervention Role (The Subject)	The Board-Mandated Override (The Top Bread)
Adaptive learning	The AI system updates its logic or "weights" based on real-time data encountered during the study	**Drift Detection**: Trigger a mandatory manual revalidation if the AI's performance deviates by more than a predefined threshold from the baseline established at protocol approval
Autonomous monitoring	The AI under study monitors animal distress, pain, or "humane endpoints"	**Veterinary Bypass**: A human veterinarian must perform physical rounds at set intervals; the AI "subject" cannot be the sole arbiter of an animal's welfare or euthanasia
Vulnerability screening	The AI identifies or screens participants based on complex, nonlinear variables	**Justice Audit**: A human ethics officer must override AI-generated participant selections if they exhibit "Algorithmic Erasure" or conflict with the Justice principles of the Belmont Report

Refer to the Master Matrix in Chapter 1 for foundational failure modes; the table defines the specific "Red Flags" that an IRB or IACUC must mandate within a protocol to ensure the investigational AI does not operate without expert human governance.

THE "BLACK BOX" AND THE TRANSPARENCY TRADEOFF

A critical limitation in reviewing AI interventions is the Opacity Paradox. The most accurate models (e.g., deep learning) are often the least explainable.

- **The Reviewer's Limit**: A board cannot "approve" a mechanism of action it cannot understand.

- **The Override Task**: As suggested by the FUTURE-AI and NIST frameworks, the board must move from *mechanistic* transparency (how it works) to *performance* transparency (how it fails). If the "Why" is a black box, the "How it fails" must be crystal clear. The human investigator must document every instance in which the AI's output was questioned, bypassed, or corrected by a human expert.

REFINING THE "THREE RS" THROUGH AI (IACUC-SPECIFIC)

In animal research, AI offers significant potential for Replacement, Reduction, and Refinement, but it introduces a "Veterinary Knowledge Gap."

1. **Refinement versus Reliability**: AI behavior monitoring can detect pain earlier than humans, but a malfunctioning AI could lead to a catastrophic failure in welfare oversight if the "human in the loop" is removed.
2. **Mechanistic Failure**: As noted in recent guidelines, AI cannot substitute for the deliberative assessment of humane endpoints. It lacks the "moral soul" to balance scientific objectives against animal distress.[15]

The Override Trigger: If a protocol proposes using AI to determine "humane endpoints" or "distress levels" without a 1:1 human veterinary backup, the IACUC must trigger a Safety Bypass. Scientific objectives can never be balanced by an algorithm; that remains a purely human ethical obligation.

- **The Skeptic's Corner**
- **Target Task**: Algorithm transparency and safety validation.
- **Adversarial Prompt**: "This AI model claims 95% accuracy. Generate five specific 'edge cases' or out-of-distribution data scenarios where this model is most likely to fail catastrophically while still reporting high confidence in its output."

PRACTICAL GUIDANCE FOR IRBS AND IACUCS

Reviewing AI-enabled research effectively requires building institutional capacity, developing structured review processes, and establishing appropriate monitoring mechanisms.

BUILDING REVIEW CAPACITY

IRBs and IACUCs need AI expertise. This means recruiting members with AI or data science backgrounds, RUAIH recommends "designated individual(s) with appropriate technology expertise, ideally in AI if available."[4] It means establishing relationships with AI experts available for consultation on technically complex protocols. It means providing training for existing members on AI fundamentals, not to make every member an AI expert but to ensure they can engage meaningfully with AI-related ethical questions and recognize when specialized consultation is needed. And it means developing processes for external expert review when internal expertise is insufficient.

STRUCTURED REVIEW FRAMEWORKS

Structured approaches support consistent review of AI protocols. RUAIH's seven elements can be adapted into an IRB review framework: Does the protocol describe appropriate AI governance structures? Are privacy protections and transparency measures adequate? Do data use agreements meet security standards? Are ongoing monitoring plans sufficient and risk-appropriate? How will AI-related safety events be captured and reported? Has bias been evaluated and will it be monitored? Will researchers and staff receive appropriate AI-specific training?

Risk stratification, categorizing AI research by risk level to guide review intensity, should follow the principle that oversight is proportionate to potential harm. Administrative AI applications with no direct participant impact require less intensive review than diagnostic AI systems making clinical recommendations. Model Card review, using standardized documentation of AI system characteristics, should become a standard part of protocol assessment.

VENDOR EVALUATION

When research uses commercial AI products, IRBs should expect protocols to address how vendors validated the tool for its intended use, whether local tuning or validation will occur, how developers evaluated bias, what monitoring tools or dashboards the vendor provides, what performance levels are guaranteed and how shortfalls are handled, and whether data use agreements adequately address permitted uses, security, and reidentification prohibition.[4]

ENHANCED CONTINUING REVIEW

AI research requires continuing review adapted to AI's dynamic nature. Performance dashboards or regular reports should give IRBs visibility into AI behavior during research. Enhanced tracking of AI-related adverse events should be standard. For adaptive systems, monitoring how the system changes over time is essential. Clear rereview triggers, significant performance degradation, detection of new biases, changes to algorithms or training data, and safety events, should be defined at initial approval, with monitoring frequency scaled to risk.

MULTIINSTITUTIONAL AI RESEARCH

AI research spanning institutions requires coordinated review approaches, potentially using single IRB arrangements, with mechanisms for sharing AI expertise across reviewing institutions, harmonized documentation and monitoring requirements, determination of whether centralized or site-based AI performance monitoring is more effective, and aligned governance structures across participating sites.

CURRENT CHALLENGES AND FUTURE DIRECTIONS

The landscape of AI ethics review continues evolving as technology outpaces frameworks. Generative AI, large language models and similar systems, creates novel risks including misinformation generation, privacy exposure from memorized training data, bias amplification, and fundamental difficulty in validating outputs whose correctness depends on context. Foundation models with diverse capabilities raise questions about how to assess systems whose potential uses extend far beyond what researchers specifically intend. Research involving multiple interacting AI systems creates complexity in predicting emergent behaviors. And real-time AI making autonomous decisions creates oversight challenges that traditional review structures weren't designed to address.

Frameworks are evolving in response. The Joint Commission and CHAI are developing detailed Responsible Use of AI Playbooks that will operationalize RUAIH's high-level guidance with specific controls and examples, and a voluntary Joint Commission Responsible Use of AI certification program is planned, potentially extending to research institutions.[4] The FDA's January 2025 draft guidance on AI-enabled devices, if finalized, will establish the most comprehensive regulatory framework for AI medical devices to date.[11] WHO and international bodies continue developing coordinated governance approaches through platforms like AIRIS.[14] And discipline-specific standards for AI research are emerging across fields.

Important research questions remain open: how to make AI involvement in research genuinely comprehensible to diverse participants, how to navigate fairness tradeoffs when different definitions of fairness conflict, which oversight approaches most effectively identify and mitigate AI risks in practice, how to translate clinical deployment governance into research contexts, and what long-term societal impacts follow from AI research and deployment. These questions will require ongoing dialogue between AI researchers, ethicists, regulators, and oversight bodies to address.

CONCLUSION

AI as a research tool, intervention, or subject of study creates ethical challenges that extend beyond traditional review frameworks while remaining grounded in traditional ethical principles. Beneficence, justice, and respect for persons still apply, but their application demands attention to algorithm transparency, bias and fairness, validation and safety, informed consent for complex technical systems, privacy risks unique to AI, regulatory classification, continuous learning hazards, adverse event detection, and animal research considerations.

Three complementary governance frameworks, RUAIH's healthcare-specific implementation guidance, FUTURE-AI's international best practices, and NIST's structured risk management approach, together provide IRBs and IACUCs with tools for evaluating AI research.[4–6] Building institutional capacity through expertise development, structured review frameworks, enhanced monitoring, consultation mechanisms, and engagement with emerging certification programs enables the rigorous oversight that AI research demands.

The goal is ensuring that AI-enabled research provides sufficient benefit to justify its risks while protecting participants, maintaining fairness, preserving privacy, and contributing to responsible AI development. As AI capabilities advance, oversight frameworks must evolve alongside them, a responsibility that falls to the research ethics community collectively and to every IRB and IACUC member individually.

The next chapter examines how AI can support participant recruitment and engagement, exploring applications that must themselves be reviewed according to the principles discussed here.

KEY TAKEAWAYS

- AI in research creates unique ethical challenges, opacity, dynamic behavior, bias, novel risk categories, and regulatory uncertainty, requiring frameworks beyond traditional IRB review.
- Three complementary governance frameworks (RUAIH, FUTURE-AI, and NIST AI RMF) provide structured approaches to evaluating AI research that IRBs can integrate.
- Algorithm transparency exists on a spectrum; IRBs should assess what level is achievable and appropriate given the AI system's role and risk level.
- Bias and fairness assessment requires evaluating AI performance across populations, choosing and justifying

appropriate fairness metrics, and planning ongoing monitoring.

- Rigorous multilayered validation (internal, external, subgroup, and local) and continuous performance monitoring during research are essential.
- Informed consent for AI research must address AI involvement, limitations, adaptability, data use, and comprehension challenges, particularly for vulnerable populations.
- Privacy protections must address AI-specific risks including reidentification, inference attacks, model inversion, and secondary data use.
- FDA's evolving regulatory framework, including the 2025 TPLC guidance, PCCP concept for adaptive algorithms, and 2026 updated CDS guidance, directly affects AI research oversight.
- Adaptive AI systems require enhanced oversight including drift detection, revalidation triggers, rollback capabilities, and participant notification protocols.
- IACUCs should evaluate how AI advances the Three Rs while ensuring adequate validation, failure protocols, and human oversight.
- Building institutional review capacity through expertise recruitment, training, structured frameworks, and consultation networks is essential.

QUESTIONS FOR REFLECTION

1. How prepared is your IRB or IACUC to review protocols involving AI systems, and what specific capacity gaps need addressing?
2. What level of algorithm explainability should be required for different types of AI research, balancing transparency needs against the potential benefits of more accurate but less interpretable approaches?
3. How can your institution ensure meaningful informed consent for AI research when technical complexity is substantial and participants may not understand the risks they face?

4. What fairness metrics and bias assessment processes are most appropriate for AI research in your institutional context, and how will you handle situations where different fairness definitions conflict?
5. How should your institution adapt RUAIH's adverse event reporting framework for research, and what AI-specific information should be captured?
6. For animal research, how can IACUCs evaluate whether AI genuinely advances the Three Rs versus introducing new risks to animal welfare?

NOTES

1. U.S. Food and Drug Administration. (2021). Artificial intelligence/machine learning (AI/ML)-based software as a medical device (SaMD) action plan. https://www.fda.gov/media/145022/download. Note: Introduced the concept of Predetermined Change Control Plans (PCCPs) to address the unique challenge of adaptive AI/ML algorithms that change after deployment, a foundational concept for understanding how regulatory frameworks accommodate AI's dynamic nature.
2. Obermeyer, Z., Powers, B., Vogeli, C., & Mullainathan, S. (2019). Dissecting racial bias in an algorithm used to manage the health of populations. *Science*, 366(6464), 447–453. https://doi.org/10.1126/science.aax2342. Note: This landmark study demonstrated that a widely used algorithm affecting millions of patients exhibited significant racial bias, reducing the number of Black patients identified for extra care by more than half, because it used healthcare costs as a proxy for health needs, and Black patients historically generated lower costs at equivalent illness levels.
3. U.S. Food and Drug Administration. (2026, January). Clinical decision support software: Guidance for industry and food and drug administration staff (updated). https://www.fda.gov/regulatory-information/search-fda-guidance-documents/clinical-decision-support-software. Note: This January 2026 update supersedes the 2022 final guidance, clarifying the scope of CDS software functions excluded from the medical device definition. Key changes include enforcement discretion for CDS producing only one clinically appropriate option, revised treatment of time-critical CDS, and updated recommendations regarding automation bias and independent review requirements.

4. Joint Commission and Coalition for Health AI (CHAI). (2025, September 17). Guidance on the responsible use of ai in healthcare (RUAIH). https://www.jointcommission.org/. Note: Establishes seven elements for responsible AI use in healthcare, with planned Playbooks to operationalize guidance and a forthcoming voluntary certification program. While designed for clinical deployment, its governance, monitoring, bias assessment, and reporting frameworks are directly adaptable to research contexts.
5. Lekadir, K., et al. (2025). FUTURE-AI: International consensus guideline for trustworthy and deployable artificial intelligence in healthcare. *BMJ*, 388, e081554. https://doi.org/10.1136/bmj-2024-081554. Note: Developed through modified Delphi consensus among 117 experts from 50 countries, providing approximately 30 best practices organized around six principles (Fairness, Universality, Traceability, Usability, Robustness, and Explainability) covering the complete AI lifecycle.
6. National Institute of Standards and Technology. (2023). Artificial intelligence risk management framework (AI RMF 1.0). NIST AI 100-1. https://www.nist.gov/itl/ai-risk-management-framework
7. Ribeiro, M. T., Singh, S., & Guestrin, C. (2016). "Why should I trust you?": Explaining the predictions of any classifier. *Proceedings of the 22nd ACM SIGKDD International Conference on Knowledge Discovery and Data Mining*, San Francisco, California USA 1135–1144. https://doi.org/10.1145/2939672.2939778. Note: Introduced LIME (Local Interpretable Model-agnostic Explanations), a widely used post hoc explainability method that provides local approximations of model behavior, enabling understanding of individual predictions without requiring global model transparency.
8. Rajkomar, A., Hardt, M., Howell, M. D., Corrado, G., & Chin, M. H. (2018). Ensuring fairness in machine learning to advance health equity. *Annals of Internal Medicine*, 169(12), 866–872. https://doi.org/10.7326/M18-1990
9. Fredrikson, M., Jha, S., & Ristenpart, T. (2015). Model inversion attacks that exploit confidence information and basic countermeasures. *Proceedings of the 22nd ACM SIGSAC Conference on Computer and Communications Security*, Denver, Colorado, 1322–1333. https://doi.org/10.1145/2810103.2813677. Note: Demonstrated that model inversion attacks can exploit confidence values revealed with predictions to reconstruct sensitive features of training data, establishing model inversion as a privacy risk category unique to machine learning systems.

10. Dwork, C., & Roth, A. (2014). The algorithmic foundations of differential privacy. *Foundations and Trends in Theoretical Computer Science*, 9(3–4), 211–407. https://doi.org/10.1561/0400000042
11. International Organization for Standardization. (2016). *ISO 13485:2016 Medical Devices, Quality Management Systems, Requirements for Regulatory Purposes.*
12. U.S. Food and Drug Administration. (2024 – update Feb 2, 2026). Medical devices: Quality system regulation amendments (QMSR). Federal Register 89 FR 7496. https://www.fda.gov/medical-devices/postmarket-requirements-devices/quality-management-system-regulation-qmsr
13. U.S. Food and Drug Administration. (2025, January 6). Draft guidance: Artificial intelligence-enabled device software functions: Lifecycle management and marketing submission recommendations. https://www.fda.gov/medical-devices/software-medical-device-samd/artificial-intelligence-software-medical-device. Note: The most comprehensive FDA guidance for AI medical devices to date, applying a Total Product Life Cycle (TPLC) approach covering model description, data lineage, performance claims, bias analysis, human–AI workflow, monitoring, and Predetermined Change Control Plans (PCCPs) for adaptive systems. With over 1,000 AI-enabled devices already authorized, this guidance has immediate practical significance.
14. World Health Organization. (2021). Ethics and governance of artificial intelligence for health. https://www.who.int/publications/i/item/9789240029200. Note: WHO's foundational guidance identifies six consensus principles for AI in health and provides governance recommendations. WHO has continued expanding this work, releasing detailed guidance on large multimodal models in March 2025 and cohosting the AIRIS 2025 conference with Korea's MFDS, which produced an outcome statement urging lifecycle, risk-proportionate governance across jurisdictions.
15. Hosseini, M., et al. (2026). Guidelines needed for the use of AI in the preparation or review of IRB, IBC, and IACUC applications. *Accountability in Research*, 8, 2612564. https://doi.org/10.1080/08989621.2025.2612564. Note: Addresses AI use across all three research oversight bodies, with particular attention to IACUC challenges including the inability of AI to assess humane endpoints, species-specific enrichment adequacy, or the ethical balance between scientific objectives and animal distress. Emphasizes that humans must remain final decision-makers in all research ethics oversight.

Part IV

Research Execution

11 AI for Participant Recruitment and Engagement

THE CHALLENGE OF RECRUITMENT AND RETENTION

Participant recruitment is the slowest part in most clinical research. The challenge is not just logistical but structural, reflecting ingrained patterns of access, trust, and representation that no technology alone can fix.

The extent of the issue is well documented. Jacques and colleagues' comprehensive review of 388 NIHR-funded randomized controlled trials found that only 53% achieved their original recruitment targets, with 30% revising their targets downward and 33% requiring recruitment extensions, figures consistent with earlier analyses spanning two decades.[1] This aligns with broader evidence: recruitment challenges are the top reason trials are discontinued or extended, affecting costs, timelines, and ultimately how quickly effective treatments reach patients.

The reach problem is equally important. Traditional recruitment methods, such as clinician referrals, posted flyers, and institutional registries, tend to identify individuals who are already well-connected to academic medical centers. This creates a self-reinforcing cycle: research samples tend to overrepresent populations with good healthcare access and underrepresent communities facing a higher disease burden. George, Duran, and Norris's systematic review documented widespread barriers to research participation among African Americans, Latinos, Asian Americans, and Pacific Islanders, including mistrust rooted in historical exploitation, lack of access to research information,

DOI 10.1201/9781003782995-15

language barriers, competing priorities, and concerns about stigma and insurance coverage.[2] These barriers are not accidental; they reflect structural inequalities that recruitment strategies need to actively address rather than unintentionally reinforce.

Eligibility screening increases the efficiency challenge. Clinical trials often involve complex sets of inclusion and exclusion criteria, such as diagnostic codes, lab results, medication histories, comorbidities, and previous treatments, which must be checked against potentially millions of patient records. Manual screening is slow, expensive, and prone to errors. Ni and colleagues demonstrated that automated eligibility prescreening using natural language processing (NLP) and machine learning can significantly improve the speed of patient identification in an emergency department, analyzing unstructured clinical text along with structured data to find candidates that manual screening might overlook.

Retention presents its own challenges aside from recruitment. Even participants who are successfully enrolled may withdraw before completing the study due to burden, adverse effects, life changes, loss of interest, or feeling disconnected from the research. Retention rates can vary greatly across studies and populations, and differential attrition can introduce bias that threatens the validity of results, even when initial enrollment was adequate and diverse.

Artificial intelligence (AI) shows real potential to address several of these challenges: efficiently screening large populations against complex eligibility criteria, identifying individuals who are likely to be interested and eligible, personalizing outreach and engagement, predicting and preventing attrition, and optimizing communication strategies. Industry benchmarks indicate AI-powered recruitment tools can increase enrollment rates by up to 65% and greatly accelerate screening cycles.[3] However, these capabilities come with risks. Without careful attention to equity, AI recruitment tools may prioritize efficiency in ways that worsen existing disparities, reaching the easiest-to-recruit populations faster while further marginalizing communities that need more targeted engagement. The ethical responsibility is to ensure AI functions as a tool for inclusion, not just a more efficient way to exclude.

PATIENT AND ADVOCACY GROUP ENGAGEMENT IN RESEARCH DESIGN

Before exploring specific AI capabilities, this chapter highlights an aspect often missing from technical discussions of AI-supported recruitment: the crucial role of patients, advocacy groups, and community partners as codesigners of research and recruitment strategies instead of just passive targets of outreach.

WHY CODESIGN MATTERS

The most technically advanced recruitment tool is useless if the research it supports is created without input from the populations it aims to serve. Studies designed with patient input are more likely to succeed in recruitment and retention because participants feel valued and understood, study procedures fit within the realities of participants' lives, consent materials address the questions participants actually have, and outcome measures reflect what matters to patients, not just what matters to investigators.[4]

Codesign is both an ethical responsibility, respecting the autonomy and expertise of affected communities, and a practical method to improve research quality and efficiency. The difference is significant: patient engagement done solely to increase enrollment risks becoming exploitative, as it reduces communities to tools rather than fostering real partnerships.

THE ROLE OF PATIENT ADVOCACY GROUPS

Patient advocacy organizations offer valuable assets to research design and recruitment: a deep understanding of their communities' priorities, concerns, and communication preferences; established trust relationships that no algorithm can replicate; practical knowledge about barriers to participation and how to overcome them; and networks capable of reaching populations invisible to institutional recruitment channels. The Patients as Partners movement, exemplified by the annual conference that gathers over 500 patient advocates, pharmaceutical executives, and regulatory professionals, has demonstrated that meaningful engagement transforms recruitment from a logistical burden into a collaborative effort.[5]

Advocacy group partnerships take many forms. Disease-specific foundations (such as the Michael J. Fox Foundation, the Cystic Fibrosis Foundation, and pancreatic cancer advocacy groups) maintain patient registries, host educational events, codevelop recruitment materials with trusted voices, and connect researchers with communities eager to participate in relevant research.[5] These partnerships succeed because they are based on reciprocity: communities contribute to research, and research provides knowledge, treatments, and infrastructure that communities value.

CODESIGNING AI RECRUITMENT TOOLS

When AI tools are incorporated into the recruitment strategy, codesign becomes even more essential. Patient advocates and community partners should participate in selecting the data used by AI tools for screening and outreach to ensure communities are comfortable with data handling. They should also review and approve AI-generated recruitment messages before they are deployed to ensure cultural appropriateness and avoid language that could cause mistrust. Additionally, they should define what "successful recruitment" means, focusing not only on enrollment numbers but also on ensuring diverse, informed, and truly voluntary participation. It is crucial to establish safeguards against algorithmic bias that could systematically exclude their communities and to evaluate recruitment experiences from the participant's perspective, rather than solely from the investigator's.

The NAACP's 2025 white paper, Building a Healthier Future: Designing AI for Health Equity, provides a framework directly applicable to AI-supported recruitment. The report promotes integrating fairness, transparency, and community involvement at every stage of health AI development, from data collection to deployment and oversight. It emphasizes that community partnerships and AI literacy are essential for building the trust and accountability necessary for equitable recruitment.[6] Its suggestions include transparency reports explaining how AI tools work, data governance councils with community representation, and community-based partnerships to ensure historically marginalized groups influence how AI is used in research affecting them.[6]

LESSONS FROM DIVERSITY-FOCUSED PROGRAMS

The NIH's All of Us Research Program provides valuable lessons on how intentional diversity design influences recruitment strategies. The program systematically identified which populations are underrepresented in biomedical research across many dimensions, including race and ethnicity, age, income, education, disability, healthcare access, and sexual and gender minorities, and then developed targeted engagement strategies for each group.[7] Importantly, All of Us partnered with community organizations and advocacy groups to create culturally appropriate engagement methods, treating communities as partners rather than just recruitment targets. The program's success in enrolling a more diverse cohort than most U.S. biomedical research shows that a diversity-focused approach works, but it requires ongoing investment in relationships, not just technology.[7]

The VA's Million Veteran Program (MVP) offers complementary lessons from a different recruitment context. Launched in 2011, MVP surpassed one million enrolled veterans in 2023, making it one of the largest genomic research programs in the world.[8] MVP's recruitment success not only illustrates what's possible when research operates within an established trust relationship, veterans already engaged with the VA healthcare system, but also demonstrates that trust alone doesn't ensure diversity. Approximately 25% of MVP participants come from minority racial and ethnic backgrounds, and the program maintains the largest cohort of Black research participants of any program worldwide. Achieving this required deliberate effort: the VA established a Diversity and Inclusion subcommittee that advised MVP's first large-scale digital outreach campaign specifically targeting women veterans, including Facebook Live events and community-amplified messaging.[9] MVP's experience shows that even within a high-trust institutional relationship, reaching underrepresented subgroups requires intentional, community-informed strategies, precisely the kind of targeted outreach that AI tools can help identify and optimize, but cannot replace.

AI tools should be built to promote this kind of intentional diversity infrastructure, signaling when enrollment demographics deviate from targets, highlighting communities that have not yet been reached, and aiding investigators in understanding why some populations are underrepresented. However, the tools must operate within a framework of authentic community partnership, not as replacements for it.

IDENTIFYING POTENTIAL PARTICIPANTS

The primary operational challenge is identifying individuals who might be eligible and interested in participating in research.

ELECTRONIC HEALTH RECORD (EHR) SCREENING

For clinical research, EHRs offer the most comprehensive source of eligibility-related information. AI systems can analyze EHR data against study eligibility criteria, evaluating complex combinations of diagnoses, laboratory results, medications, procedures, and clinical notes that would be too time-consuming to review manually. Long-term screening, which involves continuously monitoring EHRs to identify patients who become newly eligible as their conditions or treatments change, enables recruitment based on disease progression rather than snapshots taken at a single moment.[10] For rare condition studies, AI can scan large populations or multiple institutions to find the small number of eligible individuals who might otherwise never learn about relevant research opportunities.

More recently, Unlu and colleagues conducted the first prospective randomized clinical trial of AI-assisted eligibility screening, demonstrating that a large language model tool analyzing unstructured EHR data achieved eligibility determination 78% faster than manual chart review and nearly doubled enrollment in a heart failure trial.[11]

However, EHR-based screening raises important considerations that institutional review boards (IRBs) and investigators need to address. Data quality varies: EHR records may contain errors, missing information, and inconsistencies that impact screening accuracy. These quality issues are not randomly distributed but tend to be linked to healthcare access, creating systematic bias in who gets identified. Privacy protections require mechanisms that prevent identified patient information from being exposed to researchers until patients give their consent to contact, usually involving honest broker systems or research preparatory activities allowed under HIPAA. Additionally, clinician gatekeeping, even when well-meaning, can introduce bias if physicians differentially recommend research participation based on assumptions about patients' interest, ability, or compliance.

ADDITIONAL DATA SOURCES

Beyond EHRs, multiple data sources can support participant identification: insurance claims data containing diagnostic and procedure information, disease-specific registries, biobanks with stored samples and linked phenotypic data, and, increasingly, consumer wearable device data that might identify individuals with relevant health patterns (cardiac arrhythmias detected by smartwatches, sleep disturbances captured by fitness trackers). Each data source raises specific privacy, consent, and equity considerations. Claims data may be incomplete for uninsured populations. Registry participation itself reflects access and awareness biases. Wearable data is primarily available from populations with resources to purchase consumer health devices.

COMMUNITY-BASED IDENTIFICATION

For community-based research, identification methods must go beyond institutional data. AI analysis of geographic, demographic, and social determinants data can help identify communities likely to include eligible individuals. Social network analysis can map community structures and identify effective recruitment pathways. However, the most successful community-based identification depends on partnerships with community organizations, churches, community health centers, cultural organizations, and advocacy groups that can reach populations missing from institutional databases. AI can support these partnerships by helping identify organizations that are trusted messengers, analyzing which community channels work best for specific populations, and tracking outreach results to improve strategies. Nonetheless, the partnerships themselves require human relationship-building that no algorithm can replace.

PREDICTING RECRUITMENT SUCCESS AND RETENTION

Beyond identifying eligible individuals, predicting who is likely to enroll and stay in studies helps improve recruitment efforts, but it comes with significant ethical risks that need clear management.

ENROLLMENT PREDICTION AND ITS ETHICAL RISKS

AI can forecast enrollment likelihood based on demographic patterns, clinical features, previous research involvement, healthcare use, geographic factors (such as distance from research sites and transportation options), and communication responsiveness. These forecasts can enhance efficiency by focusing outreach efforts where they are most likely to succeed.

However, predicting enrollment based on historical patterns risks reinforcing the very disparities it aims to reduce.[9] If historical data reveals that some demographic groups enrolled at lower rates, possibly due to barriers that were never addressed, then prediction models trained on this data will assign those groups a lower likelihood of enrollment, leading to fewer recruitment efforts directed at them. This creates a self-fulfilling cycle: groups deemed less likely to enroll are never actively engaged, confirming the prediction and perpetuating their underrepresentation.

The solution is not to abandon prediction but to use it intentionally for equity. Prediction models should identify which populations face the most significant barriers to enrollment so that additional resources and tailored strategies can be directed toward them, reversing the efficiency logic that would otherwise focus recruitment on the easiest-to-reach populations.

Enrollment predictions should prompt equity-focused questions: Why is this population predicted to enroll at lower rates? What barriers contribute to that prediction? And what actions can we take to address those barriers?

RETENTION RISK PREDICTION

Predicting which enrolled participants are at risk of withdrawal allows for proactive retention efforts. Early warning signs, such as declining response rates, missed appointments, changes in communication patterns, and delayed data submissions, can be detected by AI monitoring systems, prompting outreach before disengagement leads to withdrawal. The benefit of prediction lies in timing: retention efforts are much more effective when they are implemented at the first signs of disengagement rather than after a participant has already decided to withdraw.

Like enrollment prediction, retention prediction should be used to promote equity rather than to prioritize triage. If certain populations show a higher risk of withdrawal, the appropriate response is not to recruit fewer of them (anticipating attrition) but to understand why they are withdrawing and address the underlying barriers, whether those barriers are logistical (transportation, scheduling), communicative (language, literacy), financial (inadequate compensation, lost wages), or relational (feeling disconnected from the research team, not receiving results).

RECRUITMENT STRATEGY OPTIMIZATION

AI can assist in optimizing various aspects of recruitment strategy while adhering to ethical standards.

CHANNEL EFFECTIVENESS AND MESSAGE OPTIMIZATION

Different recruitment channels such as clinician referral, direct mailing, social media, community outreach, advocacy group partnerships, and patient portals reach various populations with varying effectiveness. AI analysis can monitor which channels successfully reach target populations, match channels to specific demographic and clinical subgroups, compare cost-effectiveness, and evaluate whether the mix of channels reaches diverse populations or mainly accessible ones.

Recruitment messaging also benefits from optimization. A/B testing can determine which message framings, benefit descriptions, and calls to action are most effective. Personalization can customize messages to individual characteristics and concerns. Cultural adaptation can ensure messages resonate across diverse communities. And reading level optimization can make materials accessible to the intended audiences, a persistent problem since recruitment materials, like consent forms, are often written above their target audience's reading level.

However, message optimization requires ethical boundaries. The distinction between persuasion and manipulation is important: recruitment should inform and invite, not exploit psychological vulnerabilities or create false urgency. Optimization should not result in withholding essential information (such as risks, time commitments, or alternatives) in favor of more "effective" messages. Messages that are effective for one group may be inappropriate for others. Additionally, community partners, especially patient advocacy groups, should review and approve optimized messaging to ensure cultural appropriateness and accuracy before implementation.

Timing optimization, such as identifying when potential participants are most receptive to contact, determining the best spacing of recruitment communications, and pinpointing lifecycle moments (like diagnosis and treatment transitions) when research participation may be most relevant, can boost response rates. However, it must be balanced against the risk of reaching out during vulnerable moments when their ability to make autonomous decisions might be compromised.

PERSONALIZED ENGAGEMENT AND COMMUNICATION

Once enrolled, maintaining participant engagement involves communication strategies that respect individual preferences while keeping a connection to the research effort.

COMMUNICATION PERSONALIZATION AND AUTOMATION

Participants have different preferred communication channels (email, text, phone, and patient portal), ideal contact times, desired update frequency, and interest in study progress. AI can learn and honor these preferences, lowering the barriers caused by one-size-fits-all communication. Automated systems can handle routine messages efficiently: appointment reminders, survey invitations, data collection prompts for ecological momentary assessment or wearable-based studies, and study progress updates.

However, automation should be balanced with the human connection that keeps participants engaged. Overusing automation can make participation feel impersonal, possibly signaling to participants that they are just data points rather than valued partners. Important communications, such as addressing concerns, sharing results, and handling issues, should come from actual study staff who know the participant. Automated messages need to predict responses that require human attention and channel them appropriately, rather than creating dead ends that frustrate participants. Participants should always have easy access to a real person when they need help.

ENGAGEMENT MONITORING AND PROACTIVE INTERVENTION

AI monitoring of engagement indicators, including data completion rates, response timing, appointment attendance, and communication patterns, offers early detection of disengagement that allows for proactive intervention. The key benefit is proactivity: instead of learning weeks later that a participant has quietly stopped responding, study teams can identify signs of disengagement in real time and act before the relationship deteriorates.

CHATBOTS AND CONVERSATIONAL AI

Conversational AI can facilitate participant interactions for common questions about procedures, logistics, scheduling, and study progress, offering 24/7 availability and multilingual support that study staff cannot always provide. However, chatbot deployment requires clear boundaries: well-defined scope limitations, simple escalation pathways to human staff, transparent disclosure that participants are interacting with AI, and interfaces accessible to participants with different levels of technical skill. Chatbots should improve access, not replace the relationships that support ongoing participation.

RETENTION OPTIMIZATION

Sustaining participation throughout studies, especially long-term longitudinal research, demands ongoing effort that AI can assist with.

Predictive retention analytics detect disengagement early, flag crucial periods when withdrawal risk peaks (often around certain study milestones, seasonal patterns, or life changes), and send alerts for study teams. However, responding to these predictions requires human action: personalized outreach, problem-solving discussions, and real support for participants' evolving circumstances.

Different participants face various barriers to ongoing participation, including time constraints, transportation issues, competing demands, health changes, loss of interest, or a sense that their contributions aren't appreciated. Effective retention strategies tailor interventions to address individual obstacles, such as offering flexible schedules for those with limited time, remote options for those with transportation challenges, childcare, appropriate compensation that respects participants' time without being coercive, and meaningful updates that demonstrate how their contributions make a difference.

Study designs can be tailored to improve retention. AI-optimized visit scheduling around participant constraints, remote options for suitable study parts, low-burden alternatives that keep scientific validity, and milestone recognition that celebrates participant efforts all support ongoing engagement. The All of Us Research Program's use of personalized dashboards, health information return, and community events shows how programs can stay engaged by offering value to participants, rather than just collecting data from them.[7]

DIVERSITY AND INCLUSION IN RECRUITMENT

Achieving diverse, representative samples requires deliberate effort that surpasses good intentions; it needs a systematic infrastructure that AI can support.

DIVERSITY MONITORING AND GAP ANALYSIS

AI can systematically monitor enrollment demographics against targets based on disease prevalence, population makeup, or program-specific diversity standards. Intersectionality analysis, which examines representation across combinations of demographic factors (race × gender × age × socioeconomic status) rather than single categories, uncovers gaps that aggregate data often hides. Geographic diversity assessment evaluates whether recruitment reaches varied communities or is focused around research sites. Additionally, temporal monitoring observes how sample diversity changes during recruitment, allowing for adjustments before enrollment ends.

TARGETED STRATEGIES FOR UNDERREPRESENTED GROUPS

When diversity gaps are identified, targeted strategies must address the specific barriers each community faces, strategies best developed in partnership with community organizations and advocacy groups rather than imposed from outside. This means culturally tailored materials developed with community input, removing barriers that reflect the actual obstacles people encounter (transportation, childcare, language, and work scheduling), building trust that acknowledges and respects communities' historical experiences with research, and, fundamentally, conducting research that provides genuine value to the communities it aims to serve.

The NAACP's equity framework stresses that community engagement must be integrated at every stage, not added as an afterthought. For AI-supported recruitment, this involves partnering with community groups in designing and evaluating tools, making sure AI systems are checked for bias against the specific populations being recruited, and establishing feedback loops where community experiences with recruitment guide tool improvements.[6]

EQUITY MONITORING

Ongoing equity monitoring should evaluate whether recruitment strategies have uneven effects across populations, whether consent rates differ (indicating different levels of comfort or trust), whether retention rates vary among groups, and whether diverse populations have fair access to the benefits that research offers. These evaluations should be shared with community advisory boards and advocacy partners, not kept only within research teams.

ETHICAL CONSIDERATIONS

AI-supported recruitment and engagement present ethical challenges that demand proactive attention.

PRIVACY AND CONSENT

Using AI to identify potential participants involves navigating privacy protections that aim to balance research access with individual rights. The key question, what consent is necessary for automated screening of EHRs or other databases, depends on the regulatory framework (HIPAA research activities, institutional policies, and state laws) and the type of screening. Contact authorization, data use transparency, and effective opt-out options must be in place before any AI-supported outreach begins.

AUTONOMY AND MANIPULATION

Recruitment strategies must respect autonomous decision-making. The difference between legitimate persuasion (presenting relevant information convincingly) and manipulation (exploiting cognitive biases, creating false urgency, or using personal data to bypass rational thought) is ethically crucial, even if it is often blurry in practice.[11] Additional protections are necessary when recruiting populations with limited autonomy, but "reduced autonomy" should be understood in context (a patient newly diagnosed with a serious illness faces different autonomy considerations than someone responding to a social media ad) rather than as a strict category.

EQUITY AND JUSTICE

The justice considerations discussed in Chapter 9 apply with particular force to recruitment, where resource allocation decisions, which populations receive outreach, what barriers are addressed, and where recruitment funds go, directly determine whose participation counts. Community involvement and ongoing accountability, rather than unchecked optimization algorithms, must guide these decisions.

TRANSPARENCY AND TRUST

The transparency and accountability principles discussed in Chapter 9 apply directly to recruitment: potential participants should know when AI systems support identification and outreach, have the option to decline AI-mediated approaches, and researchers must maintain clear accountability for recruitment practices regardless of AI involvement.

CAPABILITIES AND LIMITATIONS: THE RECRUITMENT AND ENGAGEMENT AUDIT

While the Master Matrix in Chapter 1 outlines general AI strengths in Information Processing and Pattern Analysis, applying these to participant recruitment requires this book's most community-sensitive Override Protocols. Recruitment is not a data-mining exercise; it is a relationship-building one. AI can identify "eligible candidates" at a massive scale, but it cannot navigate the historical mistrust, structural barriers, or interpersonal chemistry that determine whether a person chooses to enroll in a study (Table 11.1).

TABLE 11.1
Recruitment-Specific Override Protocols

Recruitment Task	AI Execution (The "Meat")	The Human Override (The Top Bread)
Eligibility screening	Analyzing EHRs for complex criteria (lab results, ICD codes, and unstructured notes)	**Data Equity Audit:** Manually verify if the AI is missing "invisible" populations who have poor healthcare access and thus incomplete EHR records
Enrollment prediction	Forecasting who is likely to enroll based on historical demographic and geographic patterns	**Inversion Protocol:** If the AI predicts a group is "unlikely to enroll," trigger a manual resource allocation to *increase* engagement with that group rather than ignoring them
Retention monitoring	Detecting early signs of disengagement (missed appointments, declining survey responses)	**Relational Intervention:** Automation cannot fix a loss of trust. A human staff member must reach out to address the participant's evolving life circumstances
Message optimization	Using A/B testing to identify the most "effective" recruitment language and channels	**Cultural Sanity Check:** Advocacy groups must review AI-optimized messages to ensure they are culturally appropriate and don't cross the line into "undue inducement"

Refer to the Master Matrix in Chapter 1 for foundational failure modes; the table outlines the expert-level interventions required for equitable participant engagement.

THE "EFFICIENCY VERSUS EQUITY" PARADOX

A critical limitation in AI-driven recruitment is the Optimization Trap. If an algorithm is programmed to maximize "enrollment speed," it will naturally favor the easiest-to-reach populations, typically those already well-connected to academic centers.

- **The AI Limit**: AI optimizes for the *path of least resistance*. This often means reaching out to the same overrepresented groups, thereby automating and scaling historical exclusion.
- **The Human Task**: You must provide the Diversity Mandate. Use the NAACP's 2025 equity framework to audit your recruitment tools.[6] If the AI is accelerating your enrollment but narrowing your diversity, you must trigger a Manual Slowdown to reinvest in community-based partnerships.

TRUST, "BLACK-BOX" SCREENING, AND THE MATILDA EFFECT

Automated identification (like the RECTIFIER tool[12]) may be 78% faster than manual review, but it cannot:

1. **Sense Mistrust**: AI cannot detect the "unspoken" barriers, such as historical exploitation or fear of stigma, that prevent a candidate from responding to a digital prompt.
2. **Validate Unstructured Context**: While NLP can screen clinical notes, it may misinterpret the social determinants of health that make a participant "eligible" on paper but "unable" in reality (e.g., lack of transportation or childcare).
3. **Replace Advocacy**: As noted in the Patients as Partners movement, trust is the cornerstone of recruitment.[6] AI can identify *who* to talk to, but only a human partner (like an advocacy group leader) can be a *trusted messenger.*

The Override Trigger: If the AI identifies a candidate who meets all clinical criteria but whose social circumstances (revealed through human interaction) make the study burden too high, you must trigger a Participant Advocacy Bypass. You are the final judge of whether the recruitment approach is respectful of the person's autonomy; the AI is merely a search engine for their data.

- **The Skeptic's Corner**
- **Target Task**: Eligibility screening and message optimization.
- **Adversarial Prompt**: "Review this recruitment message for [Study]. Identify three ways this language could be seen as 'undue inducement' or manipulative to vulnerable populations, and list any groups that are systematically excluded by our current EHR screening parameters."

PRACTICAL IMPLEMENTATION

Implementing AI-supported recruitment effectively requires combining technology with human relationships, community partnerships, and ethical oversight.

REGULATORY AND IRB CONSIDERATIONS

AI recruitment tools require proper IRB review, covering the AI screening method, privacy protections for preconsent data access, the content and channels of AI-supported outreach, equity monitoring plans, and any use of predictive analytics. When recruiting vulnerable populations, enhanced safeguards are necessary to ensure that AI's efficiency does not override the additional protections these groups need.

HUMAN–AI COLLABORATION

As throughout this book, the most effective approach combines AI's systematic capabilities with the human relationship-building that ultimately determines whether people choose to participate.

COMMUNITY ENGAGEMENT INFRASTRUCTURE

When recruiting from specific communities, engagement infrastructure should come before AI deployment. This involves establishing genuine partnerships with community organizations prior to designing recruitment tools, obtaining community input on recruitment methods before applying them, ensuring AI-supported recruitment aligns with cultural norms and values as defined by the communities, structuring benefit-sharing so communities benefit from research participation beyond the study itself, and maintaining transparency about AI's role in the recruitment process.[4,6]

CONTINUOUS EVALUATION

Recruitment strategies should be continually assessed based on multiple criteria: enrollment targets, diversity goals, participant experience (measured through feedback from those who enroll and those who decline), efficiency metrics, and equity outcomes. Results should guide ongoing improvements and be shared with community partners and advocacy groups whose communities are involved in recruitment.

LOOKING FORWARD

AI capabilities for recruitment and engagement continue to advance rapidly. Improvements in NLP enable more sophisticated EHR screening of unstructured clinical text. Predictive models are becoming more accurate for both enrollment and retention, although the equity risks of prediction increase alongside its power. Decentralized and hybrid trial designs are broadening participation by reducing geographic and logistical barriers. Multilingual AI tools are starting to address language barriers that have historically excluded çnon-English-speaking populations. Additionally, real-time adaptive strategies that adjust recruitment approaches based on ongoing effectiveness data are becoming operational.[3]

However, the most significant advances may be organizational rather than technological. The increasing recognition that patient advocacy groups and community partners must be codesigners of research, not afterthoughts in recruitment, is transforming how recruitment infrastructure is developed. The NAACP's equity framework, the All of Us and MVP programs' diversity infrastructure, the Patients as Partners movement, and PCORI's patient engagement standards all represent a move toward research that is designed with communities instead of simply conducted on them.[5–8] AI tools should be built to support this shift, providing the analytical infrastructure for truly equitable, community-partnered recruitment rather than just automating traditional methods more quickly.

The core of recruitment, building trust and relationships that encourage voluntary, informed participation, will remain fundamentally human. AI's role is to enhance that human work, making it more effective, fairer, and better informed.

CONCLUSION

Participant recruitment and retention challenge most research, with many studies failing to meet enrollment targets or adequately represent diverse populations. AI offers valuable support: efficiently screening populations for eligibility, predicting enrollment and retention, optimizing recruitment strategies, personalizing engagement, and monitoring for disengagement. These capabilities can significantly improve recruitment efficiency and, when thoughtfully designed, promote equity.

But technology alone is not enough. The most essential element in fair recruitment is real engagement with the communities whose participation is needed, through patient advocacy group partnerships, community codesign, and ongoing relationship-building that treats communities as partners rather than targets. AI tools must operate within this relational framework, not as replacements for it.

When used properly, with community partnership, ethical oversight, equity checks, and human relationship-building at the core, AI can help ensure research reaches diverse groups, that eligible people learn about relevant opportunities, and that participants stay engaged throughout studies. The goal isn't faster recruitment but better recruitment: more equitable, more informed, and more respectful of the communities that make research possible.

The next chapter discusses how AI can assist with research operations and project management, helping research teams carry out complex studies efficiently and effectively.

KEY TAKEAWAYS

- Many studies do not meet recruitment targets; AI-powered tools can significantly boost enrollment rates but must be designed with equity in mind, not just efficiency.
- Patient advocacy groups and community partners should be codesigners of AI-supported recruitment strategies, their trust, cultural knowledge, and community networks are irreplaceable assets no algorithm can mimic.
- EHR screening and other automated identification methods not only provide notable efficiency benefits but also raise privacy, data quality, and equity issues that need careful safeguards.
- Enrollment and retention prediction should be used to allocate resources toward underrepresented populations, not to focus recruitment on easily accessible groups.
- The NAACP's equity framework and All of Us program serve as models for integrating fairness, transparency, and community participation into AI-supported recruitment.
- Message and channel optimization must uphold ethical boundaries between persuasion and manipulation, with community review of AI-generated content.
- Retention demands ongoing human involvement; AI provides monitoring and alerts, but meaningful engagement comes from relationships.
- Effective implementation merges AI's analytical skills with relationship-building, community partnerships, and continuous equity monitoring.
- IRB oversight of AI recruitment tools should cover screening methods, privacy safeguards, equity monitoring, and community engagement adequacy.

QUESTIONS FOR REFLECTION

1. How do patient advocacy groups and community organizations participate in developing recruitment strategies for your research, and how can AI tools support, rather than replace, those collaborations?

2. What safeguards would prevent AI-driven enrollment predictions from perpetuating existing disparities in research participation?
3. How can your institution ensure that AI recruitment tools reach populations underrepresented in your EHR data, who may be missing precisely because they face the greatest barriers to care?
4. What is the right balance between automated communication and human interaction for keeping participants engaged, and how might that balance vary among different populations?
5. How can you involve community partners in assessing whether AI recruitment tools are functioning fairly for their communities?
6. What transparency measures are most important when AI assists in recruitment, and do potential participants have a right to know how they were identified?

NOTES

1. Jacques, R. M., Ahmed, R., Harper, J., Ranjan, A., Saeed, I., Simpson, R. M., & Walters, S. J. (2022). Recruitment, consent and retention of participants in randomised controlled trials: A review of trials published in the National Institute for Health Research (NIHR) Journals Library (1997–2020). *BMJ Open*, 12(2), e059230. https://doi.org/10.1136/bmjopen-2021-059230. Note: This comprehensive review of 388 NIHR-funded RCTs found that 53% achieved their original recruitment target overall, improving to 61% for the most recent period (2017–2020). Thirty percent revised their targets (67% downward), and 33% required recruitment extensions. This study updates and extends the widely cited findings of Sully et al. (2013) and Walters et al. (2017), confirming that recruitment shortfalls remain a persistent challenge in clinical research.
2. George, S., Duran, N., & Norris, K. A systematic review of barriers and facilitators to minority research participation among African Americans, Latinos, Asian Americans, and Pacific Islanders. *American Journal of Public Health*, 104(2), e16–31. https://doi.org/10.2105/AJPH.2013.301706. Note: Reviewed 44 articles identifying both shared barriers across groups

(mistrust, lack of information access, and competing demands) and group-specific barriers, including the legacy of the Tuskegee Study and racism for African Americans, immigration concerns for Latinos, and family-based decision-making norms for Asian Americans and Pacific Islanders.

3. Lifebit. (2026). AI clinical trial optimization guide. https://lifebit.ai/blog/ai-clinical-trial-optimization-guide-2026/. Note: Industry benchmarks report that AI-powered recruitment tools improve enrollment rates by up to 65%, identify eligible candidates three times faster than manual review, and accelerate trial timelines by 30%–50%. Automated EHR text mining for cardiovascular trials has been reported to reduce the number of patients requiring manual screening by 79.9%. These figures, while promising, largely reflect vendor-reported outcomes and should be interpreted with appropriate caution.
4. Couch Health. (2024). Patient advocacy groups and co-creation in clinical trials. https://couch.health/patient-advocacy-groups-and-co-creation-in-clinical-trials/. Note: Cocreation in clinical trials, collaboration between researchers, patients, and advocacy groups to design studies that are both scientifically rigorous and patient-centered, is both an ethical imperative (respecting patient autonomy) and a pragmatic strategy: trials designed with patient input achieve better recruitment and retention because participants feel valued and understood.
5. TrialX. (2025, March 28). AI-powered clinical trial innovations at Patients as Partners 2025: Key highlights. https://trialx.com/trialx-unveils-ai-powered-clinical-trial-innovations-at-patients-as-partners-2025-key-highlights/. Note: The 12th Annual Patients as Partners in Clinical Research conference brought together 500+ industry leaders, patient advocates, pharmaceutical executives, and regulatory professionals. Discussions highlighted advocacy group partnerships for recruitment (Michael J. Fox Foundation, Let's Win Pancreatic Cancer), bilingual support for underserved communities, AI-assisted participant matching with plain-language trial explanations, and the growing recognition that patient advocates should be strategic contributors rather than passive consultation targets.
6. NAACP & Sanofi. (2025, December). Building a healthier future: Designing AI for health equity. ACE Your Health Initiative. https://naacp.org/resources/building-healthier-future-designing-ai-health-equity. Note: This 75-page framework calls for an equity-first, human-centered approach to AI in healthcare,

warning that without intentional design, AI technologies could automate and exacerbate racial disparities. Recommendations include bias audits, transparency reports, data governance councils with community representation, community-based partnerships, and AI literacy toolkits to empower patients and providers. The NAACP is actively convening policy leaders and industry to adopt the framework.

7. Mapes, B. M., Foster, C. S., Kusnoor, S. V., Epelbaum, M. I., AuYoung, M., Jenkins, G., Lopez-Class, M., Richardson-Heron, D., Elmi, A., Surkan, K., Cronin, R. M., Wilkins, C. H., Pérez-Stable, E. J., Dishman, E., Denny, J. C., Rutter, J. L., All of Us Research Program. (2020). Diversity and inclusion for the All of US research program: A scoping review. *PLoS One*, 15(7), e0234962. https://doi.org/10.1371/journal.pone.0234962. PMID: 32609747; PMCID: PMC7329113. Note: Describes how All of Us systematically assessed underrepresentation across ten demographic dimensions, racial/ethnic minorities, age, income, education, disability, healthcare access, sexual and gender minorities, and others and developed targeted community engagement strategies in partnership with community organizations. The program's emphasis on treating communities as partners and returning health information to participants provides a model for diversity-focused recruitment infrastructure.
8. Gaziano, J. M., Concato, J., Brophy, M., Fiore, L., Pyarajan, S., Breeling, J., Whitbourne, S., Deen, J., Shannon, C., Humphries, D., Guarino, P., Aslan, M., Anderson, D., LaFleur, R., Hammond, T., Schaa, K., Moser, J., Huang, G., Muralidhar, S., Przygodzki, R., & O'Leary, T. J. (2016). Million veteran program: A mega-biobank to study genetic influences on health and disease. *Journal of Clinical Epidemiology*, 70, 214–223. https://doi.org/10.1016/j.jclinepi.2015.09.016. Note: MVP, launched in 2011, surpassed one million enrolled veterans in November 2023, making it one of the world's largest genomic research programs. Approximately 25% of participants are from minority racial and ethnic backgrounds, and MVP maintains the largest cohort of Black participants of any research program worldwide. The program integrates genetic data, survey responses, and electronic health records to power precision medicine research for veterans. Unlu, O., Varugheese, M., Shin, J., Subramaniam, S. M., Stein, D. W. J., St Laurent, J. J., Mailly, C. J., McPartlin, M. J., Wang, F., Oates, M. F., Cannon, C. P., Scirica, B.M., Wagholikar, K. B., Aronson, S. J., & Blood, A. J. (2025). Manual vs AI-assisted

prescreening for trial eligibility using large language models, a randomized clinical trial. *JAMA*, 333(12), 1084–1087. https://doi.org/10.1001/jama.2024.28047. PMID: 39960745; PMCID: PMC11833652. Note: First prospective randomized trial of AI-assisted clinical trial screening. Among 4,476 heart failure patients, the LLM-based RECTIFIER tool achieved eligibility determination significantly faster (subdistribution HR 1.78, p <0.001) and increased enrollment (subdistribution HR 1.79, p =0.04) compared to manual chart review. More than 99% of AI-screened patients were identified within 15 days versus 50 days for manual screening.

9. Whitbourne, S. B., Moser, J., Gagnon, D. R., Deen, J., Amoroso, P. J., Gakhar, A., Mutalik, P., Pyarajan, S., Fiore, L. D., & Gaziano, J. M. (2023). Creating a team to focus on diversity and inclusion in research recruitment: A case report from the VA million veteran program. *Contemporary Clinical Trials Communications,* 34, 101169. https://doi.org/10.1016/j.conctc.2023.101169. PMID: 37283816; PMCID: PMC10240317. Note: Describes the VA's establishment of a Diversity and Inclusion subcommittee that advised MVP's first large-scale digital outreach campaign targeting women veterans. Strategies included Facebook Live events, community-amplified messaging, and culturally sensitive materials, demonstrating that even within a high-trust institutional relationship, intentional diversity-focused recruitment strategies are necessary to reach underrepresented subgroups.
10. Ni, Y., et al. (2015). Automated clinical trial eligibility prescreening: Increasing the efficiency of patient identification for clinical trials in the emergency department. *Journal of the American Medical Informatics Association,* 22(1), 166–178. https://doi.org/10.1136/amiajnl-2014-002887. Epub 2014 Jul 16. PMID: 25030032; PMCID: PMC4433376. Note: Demonstrated that NLP- and machine-learning-based automated eligibility screening could successfully identify patients for clinical trials in an emergency department setting, processing both structured data and unstructured clinical text to improve identification efficiency.
11. Unlu, O., Varugheese, M., Shin, J., Subramaniam, S. M., Stein, D. W. J., St Laurent, J. J., Mailly, C. J., McPartlin, M. J., Wang, F., Oates, M. F., Cannon, C. P., Scirica, B.M., Wagholikar, K. B., Aronson, S. J., & Blood, A. J. (2025). Manual vs AI-assisted prescreening for trial eligibility using large language models - a randomized clinical trial. *JAMA*, 333(12), 1084–1087. https://doi.org/10.1001/jama.2024.28047.

12. Rajkomar, A., Hardt, M., Howell, M. D., Corrado, G., & Chin, M. H. (1990). Ensuring fairness in machine learning to advance health equity. *Annals of Internal Medicine*, 169(12), 866–872. https://doi.org/10.7326/M18-1990. Note: Examines how machine learning applications in healthcare can perpetuate or amplify existing disparities through biased training data, proxy discrimination, and optimization objectives that don't account for equity. Directly relevant to AI recruitment tools that may optimize for enrollment efficiency at the cost of diversity.

12 AI for Biomedical Research Operations and Project Management

THE CHALLENGE OF RESEARCH OPERATIONS MANAGEMENT

Research operations hold a unique position in the scientific enterprise: they are crucial to the success of every study, yet they receive much less intellectual focus than study design, methodology, or analysis. Managing a clinical trial or large-scale research project involves coordinating many interconnected activities, including participant recruitment, data collection, sample processing, equipment maintenance, regulatory compliance, team communication, sponsor reporting, and analysis, across multiple sites, time zones, and institutional cultures, all within constrained budgets, limited personnel, and tight timelines.

The complexity is significant and increasing. Multisite studies, now standard for sufficiently powered clinical trials, require coordinating activities across institutions with different systems, cultures, capabilities, and regulatory environments. Adaptive trial designs, which are becoming more popular for their scientific efficiency, add operational complexity by needing real-time data analysis and protocol adjustments during the study. Decentralized and hybrid trial models, sped up by the pandemic and maintained by patient preference, spread data collection

DOI 10.1201/9781003782995-16

across clinical sites, participant homes, and digital platforms, creating coordination challenges that traditional site-based monitoring cannot solve.

Resource constraints are widespread. Most research operates on tight budgets that leave little room for error, with personnel stretched across multiple projects and equipment shared among studies. Optimizing resource use while ensuring quality remains a constant challenge, especially as studies advance and the gap between planned and actual timelines tends to grow.

Uncertainty is inherent. Equipment fails, participants withdraw, supply chains are disrupted, key personnel leave, regulatory requirements change, and enrollment falls short of projections. Treweek and colleagues' Cochrane review of recruitment strategies found that only three of 72 evaluated interventions had high-certainty evidence of effectiveness, highlighting how much of research operations involves managing under conditions of genuine uncertainty about what will work.[1]

The documentation burden alone consumes significant resources. Research produces extensive regulatory documentation, monitoring reports, deviation records, adverse event reports, protocol amendments, and institutional compliance records. Keeping these records thorough, organized in an accessible way, and ensuring they meet changing regulatory standards is resource-intensive work that seldom appears in grant budgets but is always flagged during audits when neglected.

Artificial intelligence (AI) offers real potential to solve operational challenges: improving schedules and resource use, predicting issues before they arise, automating routine monitoring and reports, enhancing cross-site communication, ensuring real-time data quality, and keeping organized records. The clinical trials sector is shifting from pilot AI projects to full operational use, with 2025–2026 marking a transition where AI-driven protocol automation, predictive risk monitoring, and centralized analytics become standard practice instead of experimental tools.[2] Nonetheless, research management ultimately depends on human leadership, setting priorities, building relationships, solving new problems creatively, and making judgment calls when multiple demands compete. AI supports these human roles; it doesn't replace them.

THE REGULATORY CONTEXT FOR RESEARCH OPERATIONS TECHNOLOGY

Research operations increasingly rely on electronic systems, whose regulatory treatment has evolved considerably. Understanding the current regulatory framework is crucial for implementing AI operational tools in compliance.

ELECTRONIC RECORDS AND SYSTEMS

The FDA finalized its guidance on Electronic Systems, Electronic Records, and Electronic Signatures in Clinical Investigations in October 2024, superseding earlier guidance and offering the most comprehensive framework to date for digital research operations.[3] The guidance clarifies several points directly related to AI-enabled operations: Part 11 compliance is assessed when records are entered into a sponsor's electronic data capture (EDC) system, not at the initial point of capture in external systems like electronic health records (EHRs); risk-based approaches to system validation are explicitly supported; and record retention requirements apply equally whether records are electronic or paper, with the expectation that metadata and audit trails are preserved.

For AI operational tools, this guidance indicates that systems generating or processing records subject to FDA predicate rules must maintain audit trails, implement access controls, ensure data integrity, and support system validation, requirements that any AI tool used in regulated research must meet.

While the October 2024 guidance established the framework, the April 1, 2026, mandatory transition has now passed. All electronic safety reporting to the FDA must now utilize the ICH E2B(R3) standard. Operational AI tools that have not been updated to this XML-based protocol are now generating "Negative Acknowledgements" (system rejections) at the FDA's Electronic Submission Gateway.

QUALITY-BY-DESIGN AND RISK-BASED APPROACHES

The broader regulatory path, reflected in ICH E6(R3)'s quality-by-design principles and risk-based oversight, aligns well with AI's capabilities.[4] Instead of using the same level of monitoring for all study activities, risk-based approaches target oversight on what matters most for participant safety and data integrity. AI is especially good at this kind of risk stratification: analyzing multiple data streams to identify which sites, processes, and time periods pose the greatest risks and then guiding human attention accordingly.

TransCelerate BioPharma's risk-based monitoring (RBM) framework offers an industry-standard methodology that AI tools can implement.[5] The framework includes systematic risk assessment at both program and protocol levels, identification of critical data and processes, development of risk indicators with set thresholds, and an Integrated Quality Risk Management Plan that coordinates oversight across functions. AI enables this framework to be practical at scale by continuously analyzing operational data streams such as enrollment rates, query response times, protocol deviation patterns, and data completeness metrics that these risk indicators rely on.

TIMELINE AND SCHEDULE OPTIMIZATION

Effective timeline management is the foundation of successful research execution and is one of the areas where AI offers the most immediate benefits.

PROJECT PLANNING AND SCHEDULING

Research project planning includes estimating activity durations, identifying dependencies, determining critical paths, allocating resources, and including buffers for uncertainty, classic project management tasks enhanced by data-driven methods.[6] AI can analyze historical data from similar studies to produce more accurate duration estimates than relying on expert intuition alone, which is especially helpful given the common tendency toward overly optimistic scheduling in research. Complex dependency networks, where the timing of one activity affects when others can start, can be optimized using computational methods that surpass manual scheduling, especially for multisite studies where site-specific capabilities and constraints add to the complexity.

Resource-constrained scheduling involves creating timelines that consider limited personnel, shared equipment, facility availability, and budget phases. It is fundamentally an optimization problem with many interrelated constraints. AI scheduling tools can find feasible schedules that balance efficiency with practical limitations, and they can identify potential resource bottlenecks that might cause delays before those delays happen.

DYNAMIC SCHEDULE ADJUSTMENT

No research timeline remains unchanged after initial contact with reality. AI's value in schedule management lies equally in its ability to adapt dynamically and in initial planning. Progress monitoring systems can compare actual completion to planned milestones, identify emerging delays through indicators such as slowing enrollment rates, increasing query volumes, and rising protocol deviation frequencies, and simulate how delays in one activity will affect subsequent dependencies. Recovery planning, which determines which schedule adjustments can regain lost time with minimal disruption, becomes more manageable with AI than through manual replanning.

For multisite studies, AI coordination tools handle the additional complexity of site-specific timelines, staggered starts, and cross-site dependencies. Balancing workload across sites by moving activities to sites with available capacity when other sites face delays can keep the overall study on track even if individual sites fall behind.

RESOURCE ALLOCATION AND OPTIMIZATION

Research resources, personnel, equipment, budget, and facilities are always limited, making allocation decisions critical for both study success and team sustainability.

PERSONNEL AND WORKLOAD MANAGEMENT

AI workforce management tools can distribute workloads evenly among team members by matching tasks to their skills and experience, preventing overload that can cause errors and burnout. Capacity planning throughout the research process, forecasting when staffing needs will peak and when cross-training or temporary support will be required, helps avoid the crisis-mode staffing common in many research operations. Scheduling optimization that balances work–life harmony with study requirements reflects an increasing understanding that maintaining a sustainable pace, rather than pushing for maximum output, leads to better long-term results in both research quality and team well-being.

EQUIPMENT, FACILITIES, AND SUPPLY CHAIN

Research equipment and facilities are costly shared resources. AI utilization optimization can schedule access to maximize throughput, coordinate preventive maintenance to reduce disruptions, resolve scheduling conflicts when multiple studies compete for limited resources, and predict future capacity needs to guide investment decisions. Supply chain management benefits from AI's ability to monitor multiple signals at once and respond to patterns more quickly than manual oversight, helping maintain adequate inventory without excess, anticipate disruptions, and identify alternative suppliers.

BUDGET MANAGEMENT

Budget management in research is often reactive, discovering issues after they become urgent. AI budget analytics shift this toward predictive management: monitoring spending against plans, analyzing burn rates to forecast depletion, identifying why actual spending diverges from projections, and suggesting reallocations when priorities shift. For multiyear grants with complex cost categories, AI forecasting that combines study progress with spending patterns provides early warnings that enable course correction instead of crisis management.

RISK MANAGEMENT AND MITIGATION

Proactive risk management separates well-run studies from those that cycle through crises. AI's pattern recognition abilities are especially useful here, shifting risk management from occasional manual checks to ongoing, data-based monitoring.

FROM PERIODIC TO CONTINUOUS RISK ASSESSMENT

Traditional risk management in research involves periodic assessments, usually at the start of a study and during monitoring visits, that identify risks, estimate their likelihood and potential impact, and develop mitigation strategies. Although this method is systematic, it has a fundamental limitation: risks develop continuously, but assessments happen only at specific times. Problems that arise between assessments might not be recognized until after they have already caused harm.

AI facilitates ongoing risk evaluation by monitoring operational data streams in real time and identifying emerging risks as they happen. The NIST AI Risk Management Framework's Map and Measure functions offer structured methods for this process: the Map function helps research teams understand the full scope of operational risks, what could go wrong, who would be affected, and the potential consequences, while the Measure function offers guidance on tracking metrics and determining whether risks are occurring.[7] Research teams can customize these functions to develop systematic risk management processes that operate continuously rather than at specific moments.

THE CLINICAL CONTROL TOWER CONCEPT

An emerging approach for AI-enabled research operations is the "Clinical Control Tower," a centralized platform that oversees operations by integrating real-time data from various sources (EDC systems, laboratory systems, site monitoring reports, enrollment trackers, and supply chain data) with predictive AI analytics. This provides a comprehensive, continuously updated view of study health.[2] This idea, increasingly discussed at industry conferences and adopted by large sponsors and CROs, marks a shift from reactive management (responding to problems after they're reported) to predictive management (anticipating problems before they occur).

Clinical Control Towers use predictive risk scoring at the site level, combining enrollment performance, data quality metrics, protocol deviation rates, query response times, and other indicators to identify sites at risk of issues before they occur. This allows targeted intervention: deploying monitoring resources, training, or support to the sites that need it most, rather than applying uniform oversight across all sites regardless of risk profile.

The tower's dashboard must now include a "Protocol Version and Standard Compliance" tile that specifically flags any data streams still using pre-April 2026 legacy formats.

SPECIFIC RISK CATEGORIES

Research encounters predictable categories of operational risk, each of which can be monitored with AI support. Recruitment risks, such as predicting enrollment shortfalls based on site activation timelines, screening-to-enrollment ratios, and competitive landscape analysis, allow for strategic interventions (like adding more sites, expanding eligibility, or increasing outreach) before delays become irrecoverable. Data quality risks, including detecting patterns of errors, missing data, or protocol deviations that indicate systemic problems rather than random issues, prompt corrective actions before data integrity is compromised.

Compliance risks, through pattern analysis of monitoring data, help identify potential Good Clinical Practice (GCP) violations, enabling remediation before regulatory findings occur. Additionally, financial risks, such as projecting budget performance based on operational trends, prevent the unpleasant surprise of funds running out before the study is completed. In the current 2026 landscape, compliance risk monitoring must include a Version Audit. AI-generated protocols or safety reporting scripts often suffer from "Historical Pattern Traps," defaulting to legacy PDF or E2B(R2) formats. Today, such a default is no longer a minor deviation; "it is a critical technical failure that prevents study data from being ingested by federal systems."

COMMUNICATION, COLLABORATION, AND DOCUMENTATION

Research coordination relies on timely, accurate, and targeted communication within teams, across sites, with sponsors, regulators, and participants.

INTERNAL AND CROSS-SITE COORDINATION

AI communication tools can improve information flow by ensuring updates reach the right people without overwhelming everyone. They can also compile progress reports from various team members or sites into clear summaries, create targeted meeting agendas based on current priorities and new issues, and record decisions for institutional memory. For multisite studies, cross-site coordination platforms can gather site updates, direct escalations to suitable central team members, promote sharing of best practices across sites, and enable virtual collaboration across different time zones and organizations.

Stakeholder communication, including adapting messages for different audiences (investigators, sponsors, institutional review boards, participants, and institutional leadership), maintaining appropriate update frequencies, and ensuring regulatory and institutional reporting requirements are met on time, benefits from AI's ability to generate customized reports, track communication obligations, and prevent missed deadlines.

DOCUMENTATION MANAGEMENT

Research produces large volumes of documentation: protocols, standard operating procedures, informed consent forms, monitoring reports, deviation records, adverse event reports, correspondence, training records, and regulatory submissions. AI documentation management systems can keep organized repositories with version control, enable quick search and retrieval, ensure compliance with regulatory documentation standards, and, most importantly, capture institutional knowledge from completed studies for future research use.

The documentation burden is not just administrative; it directly impacts research quality and regulatory compliance. The FDA's 2024 electronic systems guidance stresses that thorough audit trails and metadata preservation are essential for electronic records.[3] AI systems that automatically maintain these records, instead of relying on manual documentation that might be incomplete or inconsistent, offer both efficiency and compliance advantages.

DATA QUALITY MONITORING AND MANAGEMENT

Ensuring data quality throughout studies is essential for scientific validity and regulatory approval. Traditional methods, such as periodic data cleaning, manual source document verification, and scheduled monitoring visits, detect problems only after they occur. AI enables real-time quality monitoring that identifies issues as they happen.

REAL-TIME QUALITY SURVEILLANCE

AI can continuously monitor data quality during collection by tracking completeness (whether expected data is collected on schedule), finding consistency (identifying contradictions within or across data sources), flagging range violations (values outside expected or plausible bounds), and recognizing unusual patterns that indicate systematic issues rather than random variation. This real-time surveillance shifts quality assurance from a retrospective audit to a proactive prevention approach, allowing issues to be identified and addressed before they contaminate study datasets.

Specific data quality issues that AI identifies well include recurring missing data patterns indicating collection process problems, likely transcription or entry errors, data trends pointing to protocol deviations, equipment artifacts in laboratory or imaging data, and variations in performance across sites, time periods, or data collectors that indicate training needs or process improvements. Comparing data across sites is especially useful for multisite studies, where centralized AI monitoring can find site-level quality outliers that local oversight might miss.

WORKFLOW OPTIMIZATION

Data management workflows, from initial capture through cleaning, query resolution, locking, and analysis, have bottlenecks and inefficiencies that AI can identify and fix. Automating routine quality checks frees data management staff for judgment-heavy tasks. Optimizing integration ensures seamless data flow between EDC systems, laboratory information systems, EHRs, and analysis platforms. And access control management, which is increasingly important as data moves across institutions and systems, maintains proper security without creating barriers to legitimate use.

PROGRESS TRACKING, REPORTING, AND PREDICTIVE ANALYTICS

Systematic progress tracking allows proactive management instead of reactive crisis response.

MILESTONE MONITORING AND KEY PERFORMANCE INDICATOR (KPI) DASHBOARDS

AI progress tracking systems monitor the completion of defined milestones and required deliverables, identify activities at risk of delay, maintain focus on critical path activities, and, often overlooked, acknowledge achievements that deserve team recognition and celebration. KPI dashboards display operational metrics clearly, enabling trend analysis, benchmark comparison, and detection of anomalies that prompt investigation before issues escalate.

Automated reporting lessens the administrative workload that takes up a large part of research management time. Routine progress reports, tailored for different audiences and purposes, can be generated automatically from operational data. Exception reporting, which emphasizes only the items needing attention, directs human review to what matters instead of hiding important findings in routine data.

PREDICTIVE ANALYTICS

Understanding future trajectories, not just current status, is where AI provides the greatest strategic value to research management. Completion prediction, which estimates when studies will finish based on current operational trends, informs resource planning and stakeholder expectations. Enrollment forecasting, which predicts final sample size and enrollment timelines based on current recruitment performance, supports timely decisions about whether additional sites or strategy adjustments are necessary. Budget projection combines spending patterns with study progress to forecast financial outcomes. Additionally, risk trajectory analysis, which monitors how the risk profile evolves over time, enables strategic rather than reactive risk management.

Industry analysis indicates that AI-powered predictive analytics can shorten trial timelines by 30–50%, with predictive models reaching about 85% accuracy in forecasting trial outcomes.[8] While these numbers, mainly based on vendor-reported results, should be viewed with some caution, they demonstrate a real capability: data-driven predictions consistently outperform expert intuition in operational forecasting, especially in complex multisite studies where the number of interacting variables surpasses human cognitive capacity.

CHANGE MANAGEMENT AND ADAPTATION

Research studies rarely go exactly as planned. Protocol changes, adaptive design choices, and unexpected events all need careful handling.

PROTOCOL MODIFICATION MANAGEMENT

Protocol amendments are among the most common and significant changes in clinical research. They require tracking, impact analysis, coordinated implementation across sites and team members, identification of training needs, and comprehensive documentation updates. AI systems can manage this workflow efficiently: monitoring all modifications from submission through approval and implementation, analyzing how changes impact timelines, resources, and participant obligations, coordinating implementation across sites, and ensuring all documentation reflects the current protocol versions.

ADAPTIVE STUDY MANAGEMENT

Adaptive trial designs, which involve preplanned modifications to study parameters based on accumulating data, require operational systems capable of processing interim analyses, assessing whether prespecified decision criteria are met, simulating potential outcomes of different adaptation decisions, and coordinating stakeholder decision-making regarding adaptations. AI supports each of these functions, although the final decisions, such as whether to expand a promising treatment arm, drop a futile one, or modify eligibility criteria, remain with the study team and data monitoring committee.

RESPONDING TO UNEXPECTED EVENTS

Beyond planned changes, studies encounter truly unexpected challenges such as equipment failures, site closures, supply disruptions, public health emergencies, and key personnel departures. AI's role here is mainly to increase speed: quickly identifying the scope and impact of problems, modeling response options, providing decision-relevant information, and monitoring the implementation and effectiveness of chosen responses. The decision about what actions to take remains human; AI speeds up the gathering and analysis of information that informs that decision.

TECHNOLOGY INTEGRATION AND MANAGEMENT

Modern research operations rely on multiple technology platforms, including EDC systems, laboratory information management systems, EHRs, communication platforms, document management systems, clinical trial management systems, and randomization and trial supply management platforms, which must work together.

AI can optimize this technology ecosystem by ensuring smooth data flow between systems, monitoring system performance and availability, detecting errors or malfunctions, managing appropriate access controls, and maintaining audit trails and compliance documentation that regulatory requirements demand.[3] Security monitoring, identifying threats or unauthorized access attempts, is increasingly important as research data flows across institutional boundaries and cloud platforms.

The integration challenge is especially severe for decentralized trials, where data comes from participant devices, remote monitoring platforms, local laboratories, and electronic patient-reported outcome systems, in addition to traditional site-based collection. AI middleware that normalizes, validates, and routes data from various sources, while keeping the audit trails and metadata intact as required by the regulatory framework, is becoming essential infrastructure rather than just an optional enhancement.

PRACTICAL IMPLEMENTATION

Implementing AI for research operations involves balancing the real benefits of automation and analytics with the organizational change management needed for any technology deployment.

TOOL SELECTION AND INTEGRATION

The expanding market for AI-enabled research management tools demands careful evaluation: identifying specific operational challenges worth tackling, comparing available tools to institutional needs and limitations, ensuring seamless integration with existing systems and workflows, prioritizing user-friendly interfaces suited for research staff (who may not be tech experts), and assessing vendors' reliability, support capabilities, and long-term stability. Following the phased approach described in Chapter 1, implementation should start with high-value, low-risk applications like automated reporting and quality monitoring before moving to predictive risk management and adaptive scheduling.

BALANCING AUTOMATION AND HUMAN JUDGMENT

The human–AI collaboration principles discussed in Chapter 9 apply directly to operations. Override capabilities, allowing managers to deviate from AI recommendations when context warrants, must be straightforward and culturally normalized rather than treated as exceptional.

To move beyond high-level policy and truly "normalize" the act of overriding AI, institutions should implement formal Verification Protocols. These protocols explicitly define which AI outputs require manual validation and the specific methods for performing that validation. By codifying these steps, the "override" is no longer seen as a lack of trust in the technology but as a standard operating procedure for maintaining scientific integrity.

The goal is not to replicate 100% of the AI's work, which would negate the efficiency gains, but to use statistically sound sampling and targeted expert review to maintain the "Human–AI–Human" sandwich throughout the study's operational phase.

This oversight structure is designed to fulfill the "Quality by Design" requirements outlined in ICH E8(R1) and the monitoring standards of Responsible Use of AI in Healthcare Element 4.

Escalation protocols should clearly define when issues require human attention, preventing both dangerous autonomy, AI making consequential decisions without human review, and alert fatigue, humans overwhelmed by trivial escalations.

CHANGE MANAGEMENT AND TEAM ENGAGEMENT

Technology implementation fails when it alienates the people it's meant to serve. Engaging stakeholders by involving team members in tool selection and workflow design fosters ownership. Providing comprehensive training ensures competence and confidence. Regular feedback collection helps identify issues before frustration builds up. Additionally, paying close attention to how AI tools influence team dynamics, ensuring monitoring capabilities don't turn into oppressive surveillance, workload adjustments focus on sustainable pacing rather than maximum output, and technology supports rather than replaces personal connections, determines whether implementation succeeds or stalls.

CAPABILITIES AND LIMITATIONS: THE OPERATIONAL AUDIT

While the Master Matrix in Chapter 1 outlines general AI strengths in Oversight Tasks and Resource Allocation, applying these to biomedical research operations requires a specific set of Operational Override Triggers. AI can optimize a schedule or flag a data outlier, but it cannot navigate the institutional politics, staff burnout, or "messy" clinical realities that determine a study's success.

As established in the Verification Protocol (Table 12.1), efficiency gains in the "Execution" phase must be reinvested into a human-led audit of the AI's logic (Table 12.2).

THE "OPTIMISM BIAS" AND ALGORITHMIC RIGIDITY

A critical limitation in AI-led project management is the Historical Pattern Trap. AI forecasts are based on past performance data that may not account for the "Black Swan" events of

TABLE 12.1
Example Verification Protocol for AI-Assisted Biomedical Research

AI Research Task/Output	Potential Risk/ Failure Mode	Human Validation Step (Verification Protocol)
Automated participant screening	"False negatives" (eligible patients incorrectly excluded by AI)	Manual audit of a randomized 10% sample of all AI-excluded candidates to ensure no eligible participants were missed
Literature synthesis/ evidence mapping	"Hallucinated" citations or omission of key contradictory studies	Cross-reference every AI-cited "key finding" against the primary source PDF; perform a manual "sanity check" search in PubMed for known seminal authors in that niche
Data cleaning and outlier detection	AI incorrectly flagging valid clinical extremes as "errors" or noise	Expert clinical review of all data points flagged for removal to confirm they are physiologically impossible rather than rare clinical presentations
Informed consent form generation	Omission of site-specific risk language or use of overly complex "AI-speak"	Mandatory line-by-line review by the Study Coordinator to ensure all IRB-approved "must-have" risk clauses are present and at the correct reading level
Statistical code generation (R/Python)	Subtle logic errors in data transformation (e.g., miscalculating time-to-event)	Independent "code-review" or "shadow-coding" where a human statistician manually recalculates a subset of the primary outcome metrics

2026, such as sudden shifts in FDA guidance (e.g., the October 2024 Electronic Systems update[3]) or global supply chain disruptions.

- **The AI Limit**: AI assumes a level of consistency that rarely exists in a multisite clinical trial. It cannot "feel" the mounting frustration of a research team or the declining morale at a struggling site. For example, an

TABLE 12.2
Operations-Specific Override Protocols

Operational Task	AI Execution (The "Meat")	The Human Override (The Top Bread)
Schedule optimization	Analyzing dependencies to create a "mathematically perfect" study timeline	**Plausibility Audit:** Manually adjust for "unwritten" delays, such as local holiday slowdowns, typical IRB turnaround times, or known equipment maintenance cycles
Predictive risk scoring	Flagging clinical sites at risk of failure based on enrollment and query rates	**Root Cause Intervention:** AI identifies the *what*; humans must find the *why*. Determine if a site is "failing" due to poor training or an unavoidable local patient surge
Real-time quality monitoring	Automatically flagging data points that fall outside plausible clinical ranges	**Clinical Sanity Check:** Verify that a "violation" isn't actually a rare but valid clinical presentation. AI tends to "clean" away the most interesting (and real) data outliers
Budget burn tracking	Forecasting fund depletion based on current operational speed and recruitment	**Strategic Reallocation:** Humans must decide which study arms to prioritize if funds run low. AI can project a deficit, but it cannot make a value-based decision on study futility

Refer to the Master Matrix in Chapter 1 for foundational failure modes; the table defines the expert-level interventions required for study management.

AI trained on 2025 data will suggest safety reporting workflows that are now obsolete as of the April 1, 2026 E2B(R3) mandate.

- **The Human Task**: You must provide the Interpersonal Intervention. Use AI to identify the "sites of concern." The Human Task is to perform a "Regulatory Stress Test" on all AI-suggested operational outputs to ensure they haven't fallen into the 2026 Black Swan trap of obsolete standards.

DATA QUALITY VERSUS DATA SANITIZATION

While AI is 85% accurate in forecasting trial outcomes,[8] its "Quality Monitoring" can lead to Over-Cleaning:

1. **Erasing the Extremes**: In its attempt to identify "errors," AI may flag valid, extreme physiological values as "noise," potentially masking a rare adverse event or a significant treatment effect.
2. **Audit Trail Fragility**: While AI can automate documentation, the human investigator remains legally accountable for the Data Provenance. As required by FDA Part 11 and ICH E6(R3),[4] the "Accountability Sign-off" must be a conscious human act, not an automated timestamp.

The Override Trigger: If the AI suggests a study timeline or a RBM plan that ignores the "human variables" of your specific team (e.g., a key staff departure or a site-specific infrastructure gap), you must trigger a Management Bypass. You are the final arbiter of operational feasibility; the AI is merely the clerk tracking the metrics.

THE SKEPTIC'S CORNER

- **Target Task**: Safety Reporting and Regulatory Compliance.
- **Adversarial Prompt**: "This AI-generated safety protocol was drafted using a 2025 template. Identify where it still refers to 'voluntary' E2B(R3) adoption. Rewrite the automated submission logic to acknowledge the April 1, 2026, mandatory cutoff, and flag any legacy 'R2' data fields that will now trigger a system-level rejection at the FDA gateway."

ETHICAL CONSIDERATIONS

AI-supported research operations raise ethical issues that enthusiasm for implementation can hide.

PRIVACY, SURVEILLANCE, AND AUTONOMY

Operational monitoring systems that track data entry patterns, response times, error rates, and work schedules generate information about individual performance that could be used oppressively. Proportionate monitoring, which collects only data necessary for legitimate management purposes, is an ethical requirement, not just a best practice. Team members should be informed of what is monitored and how that information is used. The line between productive oversight (ensuring study quality) and surveillance (controlling team behavior) must be maintained through clear policy and practice.

EQUITY AND WELL-BEING

AI optimization tools should prioritize team well-being as well as operational efficiency. Workload balancing must aim for reasonable schedules, not maximum output. Resource distribution among team members and sites should be fair. Scheduling should consider work–life balance. If AI systems can detect disengagement patterns in participants, they should also identify overload patterns in staff and trigger supportive interventions instead of just performance management. Sustainable research operations lead to better science than exhausted teams working at full capacity.

ACCOUNTABILITY

AI decision support does not lessen management accountability. When operational decisions rely on AI analytics for resource allocation, scheduling, or risk prioritization, the manager who acts on those analytics remains responsible for the results. The transparency and error-correction principles discussed in Chapter 9 apply here, with particular attention to maintaining trust among team members, sponsors, and regulators who need to understand AI's role in operational decisions.

LOOKING FORWARD

Research operations AI is shifting from standalone tools to integrated ecosystems. The Clinical Control Tower concept, which offers centralized, predictive, and comprehensive oversight, exemplifies this trend: AI that not only supports individual tasks but also provides a continuous, overall view of study health across all operational areas.[2] Natural language interfaces are making operational tools more user-friendly for nontechnical users. Predictive capabilities are advancing with larger training datasets and more advanced models. Additionally, the regulatory environment is evolving, with ICH E6(R3)'s quality-by-design principles, the FDA's updated electronic systems guidance, and European Medicines Agency's focus on risk-based oversight creating a regulatory landscape that supports rather than hinders AI-enabled operations.[3,4]

However, two warnings are necessary. First, operational AI is only as effective as the data it processes, and research operations data is often scattered across systems, inconsistently organized, and variably complete. Integration and data quality are essential for AI to be valuable, not afterthoughts. Second, the efficiency gains AI offers should be reinvested into research quality and team sustainability, rather than simply used to do more with less, which only deepens the resource scarcity that makes research operations difficult in the first place.

The core aspects of research management, leading teams, making tough decisions amid uncertainty, building collaborative relationships, and maintaining morale through setbacks, will always be human endeavors. AI enhances this human work, making it more informed, efficient, and proactive. The aim isn't algorithmic management but augmented leadership: human judgment supported by comprehensive analytics, human decision-making guided by predictive insights, and human relationships maintained with less administrative burden.

CONCLUSION

Research operations and project management involve coordinating complex, interdependent activities with limited resources under conditions of real uncertainty. AI provides significant support: optimizing schedules and resource allocation, enabling ongoing rather than periodic risk management, automating routine monitoring and reporting, facilitating cross-site communication, ensuring real-time data quality, tracking progress predictively, and maintaining comprehensive documentation.

These capabilities are becoming an operational reality. AI-powered protocol automation, predictive risk monitoring, centralized analytics, and quality-by-design workflows are transitioning from pilot projects to standard practice, a shift driven by both technological advancement and a regulatory environment that increasingly supports risk-based, technology-enabled oversight.

But operational tools only succeed when they serve the people using them. Implementation that emphasizes team engagement, preserves human judgment, respects work–life balance, and maintains transparency about AI's role leads to sustainable operational improvements. Implementation that focuses on maximizing extraction at the expense of well-being results in short-term efficiency gains but causes long-term organizational harm.

The next chapter discusses how AI can assist with data collection and management, including the emerging field of synthetic data generation and augmentation.

KEY TAKEAWAYS

- Research operations face increasing complexity from multisite designs, adaptive protocols, decentralized trials, and expanding regulatory requirements, and AI helps manage this complexity systematically.
- The FDA's October 2024 electronic systems guidance and ICH E6(R3)'s quality-by-design principles establish a regulatory framework that supports AI-enabled operations while enforcing audit trails, validation, and data integrity.
- AI analysis of dependencies, historical patterns, resource constraints, and real-time progress enhances timeline and schedule optimization, especially for multisite studies.

- RBM, implemented through frameworks like TransCelerate's RBM methodology, shifts with AI from periodic manual assessments to continuous, predictive surveillance.
- The Clinical Control Tower concept, a centralized, AI-integrated operational oversight system, represents the emerging paradigm for managing research operations.
- Data quality monitoring changes from retrospective auditing to real-time surveillance, identifying issues as they happen rather than after they've contaminated datasets.
- Predictive analytics for enrollment, completion, budget, and risk trajectories enable proactive management instead of reactive.
- Ethical implementation demands proportional monitoring, workload fairness, a sustainable pace, transparency, and maintained human accountability.
- Operational AI is only as effective as its data; integration and data quality are essential for generating value.

QUESTIONS FOR REFLECTION

1. What operational challenges in your research take up the most management time, and which are easiest to support with AI without sacrificing quality or team dynamics?
2. How can RBM, supported by AI analytics, improve oversight efficiency while maintaining or even enhancing participant safety and data integrity?
3. What balance between operational efficiency and team well-being should inform AI implementation decisions in your research environment?
4. How ready is your institution's technology infrastructure for the integration required by AI operational tools, and what investments in data quality are needed initially?
5. What transparency measures should be used to keep team trust while implementing AI monitoring and optimization tools?

NOTES

1. Treweek, S., Pitkethly, M., Cook, J., Fraser, C., Mitchell, E., Sullivan, F., Jackson, C., Taskila, T. K., & Gardner, H. (2018). Strategies to improve recruitment to randomised trials. *Cochrane Database of Systematic Reviews*, 2, MR000013. https://doi.org/10.1002/14651858.MR000013.pub6. Note: This landmark Cochrane review evaluated 72 comparisons of recruitment strategies. Only three had high-certainty evidence: open trials improve recruitment over blinded trials (absolute improvement 10%), telephone reminders to postal nonresponders improve recruitment (absolute improvement 6%), and a specialized participant information leaflet development approach had no effect. The finding that so few strategies have strong evidence underscores the uncertainty inherent in recruitment operations.
2. Merative. (2026, February). Trends for 2026: Targeted AI, continuous trials, and navigating uncertainty. https://www.merative.com/blog/clinical-trial-trends-2026. Note: Industry analysis documenting the transition from AI pilot projects to operational implementation in clinical trials, with AI-powered protocol automation, predictive risk monitoring, and centralized analytics becoming standard practice. The concept of the Clinical Control Tower, integrating real-time operational data with predictive AI insights, is increasingly adopted for comprehensive trial oversight.
3. U.S. Food and Drug Administration. (2024, October). Electronic systems, electronic records, and electronic signatures in clinical investigations: Questions and answers, Guidance for industry. https://www.fda.gov/regulatory-information/search-fda-guidance-documents/electronic-systems-electronic-records-and-electronic-signatures-clinical-investigations-questions. Note: This October 2024 final guidance supersedes the 2017 draft guidance and earlier documents. Key provisions clarify that Part 11 compliance is assessed at entry into a sponsor's EDC system (not at original capture in external systems like EHRs), that risk-based approaches to system validation are acceptable, and that metadata and audit trails must be preserved regardless of record format. Directly applicable to AI operational tools processing regulated research data.
4. International Council for Harmonisation. (2023). ICH E6(R3): Good clinical practice, principles and overarching requirements (Step 2 draft). https://www.ich.org/page/efficacy-guidelines. Note: The major revision of the GCP guideline introduces quality-by-design principles, risk-proportionate monitoring

approaches, and explicit recognition of evolving technology in clinical research. Its emphasis on identifying critical-to-quality factors and applying oversight proportionate to risk aligns with AI-enabled risk-based monitoring approaches.

5. TransCelerate BioPharma. (2013–present). Risk-based monitoring initiative. https://www.transceleratebiopharmainc.com/initiatives/risk-based-monitoring/. Note: TransCelerate's RBM methodology, developed by a consortium of major pharmaceutical companies, provides model guidelines for targeted, risk-based monitoring applicable to any size organization and any trial phase. Key tools include the Risk Assessment and Categorization Tool (RACT) and the Integrated Quality Risk Management Plan (IQRMP). AI operationalizes this framework by continuously processing the operational data streams that risk indicators depend on.
6. Heldman, K. (2018). *Project Management JumpStart* (4th ed.). Sybex. Note: Provides foundational project management concepts, activity sequencing, critical path analysis, resource-constrained scheduling, risk identification, and stakeholder communication, applicable to research operations. Aligned with the Project Management Body of Knowledge (PMBOK Guide, 6th edition).
7. National Institute of Standards and Technology. (2023). Artificial intelligence risk management framework (AI RMF 1.0). NIST AI 100-1. https://www.nist.gov/itl/ai-risk-management-framework. Note: The four-function framework (Govern, Map, Measure, and Manage) provides structured approaches to AI risk management applicable to research operations. The Map function helps teams understand operational risk contexts; the Measure function guides metrics tracking; the Manage function directs mitigation resources. Research teams can adapt these functions for systematic operational risk management.
8. Lifebit. (2026). AI clinical trial optimization guide. https://lifebit.ai/blog/ai-clinical-trial-optimization-guide-2026/. Note: Industry benchmarks reporting AI-powered tools accelerating trial timelines by 30%–50%, improving patient recruitment rates by 65%, achieving 85% accuracy in forecasting trial outcomes, and enabling real-time safety monitoring with 90% sensitivity for adverse events. These figures are largely vendor-reported and should be interpreted with appropriate caution, but they reflect real capabilities in data-driven operational prediction.

Part V

Data and Analysis

13 Data Collection and Management

THE CHALLENGE OF RESEARCH DATA IN THE ARTIFICIAL INTELLIGENCE (AI) ERA

Research data has changed in nature, not just size. Genomic studies now generate terabytes of sequencing data per experiment. Clinical trials with continuous wearable monitoring produce millions of data points per participant over months or years. Social and behavioral science research uses large digital trace datasets, social media activity, mobile phone records, and web behavior, far surpassing what previous generations could access. Traditional manual methods for data collection and management simply cannot keep up with these demands.

Volume is just one part of the challenge. Research data comes in many forms, including structured databases, unstructured clinical notes, medical images, audio files, video, sensor streams, and increasingly complex combinations, all from different institutions with varying systems, terminologies, and quality standards. Combining these diverse sources while preserving quality and consistency calls for methods that go beyond what manual processing can reliably accomplish.

Quality is the most important factor. Research validity relies entirely on data quality; errors, inconsistencies, missing values, and systematic biases spread through analyses and weaken conclusions, no matter how advanced the methods are. The Good Machine Learning Practice (GMLP) principles, originally issued jointly by the FDA, Health Canada, and the UK MHRA in 2021 and finalized as an international standard by the International Medical Device Regulators Forum (IMDRF) in January 2025, emphasize this point: AI and machine learning systems are "only as good as the data used to train them," making data quality

DOI 10.1201/9781003782995-18

essential for every subsequent application.[1] Poor data leads to not only incorrect answers but also confidently wrong answers when processed by powerful AI tools that lack the contextual judgment to detect problems humans would notice.

The reproducibility requirement adds another layer of complexity. Scientific credibility relies on other researchers being able to understand, evaluate, and reproduce data collection and processing methods. The FUTURE-AI international consensus framework highlights traceability, which involves keeping detailed records that ensure reproducibility and accountability, as one of six key principles for trustworthy AI in healthcare.[2] Without thorough provenance documentation, even the most rigorous data collection becomes a black box that others cannot scrutinize.

Multisite coordination, regulatory compliance (privacy laws, institutional policies, and ethical standards), consent management, deidentification, access controls, audit trails, and long-term stewardship all contribute to a complex data management landscape. AI-assisted data collection and management are becoming essential, not just convenient, for modern large-scale research.

FOUNDATIONAL FRAMEWORKS FOR AI IN DATA MANAGEMENT

The governance frameworks introduced in earlier chapters each address distinct aspects of data management; here, I focus on the specific principles most relevant to data quality, documentation, and stewardship. Several frameworks offer structured guidance for responsible AI use in research data management. Instead of viewing these as checklists, researchers should understand how each framework tackles different parts of the data lifecycle.

GMLP PRINCIPLES

The ten GMLP guiding principles, finalized by the IMDRF in January 2025 and building on the original 2021 FDA/Health Canada/MHRA framework, outline standards directly relevant to research data management.[1] Principle 2 emphasizes robust software engineering, medical device design, and security practices throughout the total product lifecycle, positioning data quality as fundamental rather than optional. Principle 3 focuses on representativeness: clinical evaluations must utilize datasets that accurately represent the target patient population, requiring explicit attention to demographic diversity, clinical variability, and potential sources of collection bias. Principle 5 addresses reference standards, requiring that chosen reference standards are fit-for-purpose, which influences how data is collected and curated from the outset. Principle 10 mandates that deployed models are continuously monitored for performance and retraining risks are effectively managed, emphasizing the need for data collection systems capable of detecting data drift or performance decline over time.

FUTURE-AI TRACEABILITY

The FUTURE-AI framework's traceability principle provides the most comprehensive description of what documentation standards AI data management systems should support.[2] Traceability includes thorough documentation of data sources, collection methods, preprocessing steps, and quality decisions; provenance tracking records the origin and processing history of each data element; version control monitors changes to datasets with clear versioning to enable reproducibility; and decision audit trails document exclusion criteria, imputation methods, corrections, and other judgments that influence the final dataset. For research contexts, these requirements translate into specific infrastructure needs: data management systems must not only store data but also maintain the full lineage that allows other researchers to understand how the data reached its final form.

NIST AI RMF MAP FUNCTION

The NIST AI Risk Management Framework's Map function helps organizations understand the context in which AI systems operate, and for data management, context is everything.[3] Mapping data contexts involves understanding where data originates, which populations it represents, what biases it might contain, and how it relates to its intended applications. It also includes identifying stakeholders affected by data collection and those who should be consulted about data practices. Additionally, it involves understanding what can go wrong, such as quality failures, privacy breaches, representation gaps, and security vulnerabilities, as well as evaluating the potential consequences, from minor inconveniences to significant harms impacting research validity, participant welfare, or broader populations. Applying the Map function before implementing AI data tools helps research teams anticipate and plan for risks rather than discovering them after deployment.

FAIR PRINCIPLES

The FAIR Guiding Principles, making data Findable, Accessible, Interoperable, and Reusable, established a framework for scientific data stewardship that has become foundational to open science.[4] In an AI context, FAIR compliance gains additional importance: AI systems require machine-readable metadata, standardized formats, and clear documentation to process data effectively. The FAIR^2 (FAIR Squared) extension, launched by Frontiers in March 2025, builds on the original principles by adding AI-readiness requirements, integrating data with provenance, methodology documentation, and detailed data dictionaries to create context-rich, machine-actionable datasets compatible with major AI frameworks.[5] This development reflects a growing recognition that data stewardship must serve both human researchers and the AI tools they increasingly rely on.

AI-ENHANCED DATA COLLECTION

AI transforms data collection across multiple dimensions, not only automating existing processes but also enabling entirely new ways to capture and sample data in real time.

AUTOMATED DATA CAPTURE

- **Intelligent Form Processing**: Combines optical character recognition (OCR) with natural language processing to extract structured data from paper forms, handwritten notes, and legacy unstructured documents.
- **Voice-to-Data Conversion**: Captures spoken information from clinical encounters and research interviews, transforming speech into structured data elements.
- **Computer Vision Systems**: Extract quantitative data from visual sources, such as counting cells in pathology slides, measuring features in radiology images, coding behaviors from observation videos, or classifying environmental features from photographs.
- **Sensor Data Integration**: Processes high-frequency streams from physiological monitors, environmental sensors, and motion tracking devices, extracting meaningful signals from continuous data flows.

ADAPTIVE AND INTELLIGENT SAMPLING

Beyond automating capture, AI allows for more advanced methods of selecting what data to gather. Adaptive sampling modifies collection strategies in real time based on incoming data, focusing effort where additional data offers the greatest benefit, whether in areas of high uncertainty, underrepresented groups, or emerging trends. Machine learning can determine which potential participants would best contribute to research goals based on the current sample makeup, optimizing recruitment for statistical power while reducing unnecessary enrollment burdens. Sequential experimental designs that adapt according to interim results, gathering more data on promising conditions and less on clearly ineffective ones, decrease overall data collection while maintaining or enhancing inferential power.

For studies monitoring rare events, AI can continuously oversee data streams, triggering detailed "burst" collection protocols the moment an unusual case is detected. Adaptive data collection tools that respond to participant responses, gathering detailed information when clinically relevant and reducing effort when additional detail offers little analytical benefit, can improve both data quality and participant experience at the same time.

REAL-TIME QUALITY MONITORING DURING COLLECTION

Perhaps AI's most significant contribution to data collection is enabling quality assessment at the point of capture rather than after the fact. Entry validation systems check data in real time, flagging implausible values, internal inconsistencies, or patterns indicating quality issues before data is finalized, when correction is easier rather than after the research visit has ended and the participant has left. Missing data detection identifies gaps immediately, allowing prompt follow-up while information remains accessible. Protocol compliance monitoring tracks adherence to collection procedures, flagging deviations that could impact validity. Additionally, instrument calibration tracking monitors measurement devices for drift or degradation, ensuring data quality is maintained across collection periods without the surprises that periodic manual calibration checks typically miss.

AI-POWERED DATA MANAGEMENT

Beyond collection, AI changes how data is organized, curated, documented, and maintained throughout its lifecycle.

AUTOMATED CURATION AND ENTITY RESOLUTION

Data curation, the ongoing work of organizing, cleaning, and maintaining research datasets, is labor-intensive and critically important. AI assists through intelligent categorization (automatically classifying data elements into logical structures), duplicate detection (identifying duplicate or near-duplicate records from data entry errors or system integration issues), and entity resolution (determining when records from different sources refer to the same participant, sample, or location). Entity resolution is particularly valuable in multisite studies and data integration projects where the same individual may appear in multiple datasets under slightly different identifiers, a problem that grows exponentially with the number of data sources but that AI handles far more reliably than manual matching at scale.

Anomaly flagging, identifying data points that are unusual enough to warrant human review, bridges curation and quality assurance. The key distinction here is between flagging and deciding: AI should identify anomalies for human evaluation, not automatically classify them as errors. A seemingly impossible laboratory value might be a transcription error or a genuine clinical finding, and determining which requires domain knowledge that AI does not possess.

SMART METADATA AND DOCUMENTATION

Metadata, data about data, is the infrastructure that makes research datasets discoverable, interpretable, and reusable. AI can extract metadata automatically from data content (identifying date ranges, geographic coverage, variable types, and other characteristics), add semantic annotations linking concepts to standardized vocabularies and ontologies, assist with generating data documentation (variable descriptions, codebooks, and data dictionaries), and create searchable indices enabling researchers to find relevant data across large repositories. These capabilities directly support FAIR compliance by ensuring appropriate metadata, standard formats, and clear documentation, reducing the manual documentation burden that otherwise makes FAIR aspirational rather than operational.[4]

DATA INTEGRITY AND THE QUALITY MANAGEMENT SYSTEM REGULATION (QMSR) (ISO 13485) MANDATE

As of February 2, 2026, the FDA has replaced the legacy Quality System Regulation with the QMSR. This rule harmonized 21 CFR Part 820 with the international standard ISO 13485:2016. For data management, this means AI-automated audit trails are now evaluated under a risk-based validation model. If an AI data tool does not maintain a "Total Product Life Cycle" log that meets ISO standards, study data may be deemed inadmissible during a regulatory audit.[6]

VERSION CONTROL AND PROVENANCE TRACKING

Aligned with FUTURE-AI traceability principles, AI data management systems should maintain comprehensive provenance records throughout the data lifecycle.[2] This means tracking the complete lineage of each data element, including the original source, collection method, every processing step, and every quality decision, with enough detail to reproduce any transformation. Every correction, exclusion, imputation, and modification should be logged along with the decision, the rationale, and the decision-maker. Version control should track dataset changes with clear versioning that allows any previous state to be reconstructed. When data leaves research systems, is shared with collaborators, deposited in repositories, or submitted with publications, documentation of what was exported, to whom, under what agreements, and for what purposes maintains the chain of accountability.

This level of documentation might seem burdensome, but it is exactly what reproducibility requires and what regulatory auditors look for. AI makes it possible by automatically recording data as a natural part of data operations instead of needing separate manual documentation.

DATA QUALITY ASSURANCE WITH AI

Ensuring data quality is an ongoing process, not just a single phase, throughout the research lifecycle. AI shifts quality assurance from occasional manual checks to continuous automated monitoring.

CONTINUOUS QUALITY MONITORING

AI quality monitoring works across multiple areas at the same time. Completeness checking sees if the expected data is being collected and finds systematic gaps that need fixing. Consistency validation checks logical links within and across records, chronological sequences, mathematical rules, and categorical dependencies, flagging violations that may indicate errors. Range and format verification find data entry mistakes and system problems. Cross-source validation compares information from different data sources that gather similar data, spotting discrepancies that need to be resolved. Additionally, temporal pattern analysis studies how data changes over time, detecting unexpected shifts that could signal quality issues rather than real changes.

ANOMALY AND OUTLIER DETECTION

AI anomaly detection goes beyond simple range checking. Statistical outlier detection identifies values significantly deviating from expected distributions. Pattern-based detection learns normal data patterns and spots deviations that basic statistical methods miss. Contextual detection evaluates values in context; a blood pressure reading that is normal alone but unusual for a specific patient needs a domain-aware assessment. Collective detection finds groups of observations that are unusual together, even if individual values seem normal, which helps catch systematic issues. Temporal detection recognizes unusual patterns over time, such as sudden shifts, unexpected trends, cyclical anomalies, and other patterns that may indicate quality concerns or genuine phenomena requiring documentation.

The key insight is that anomaly detection suggests candidates for human review, not final decisions. The difference between an error and a real outlier, or between a value that should be fixed and one that needs further investigation, depends on human expertise that AI cannot provide. AI's role is to guide human focus effectively: reviewing every data point is impossible, but examining the ones flagged as unusual by AI is feasible and valuable.

PREDICTIVE QUALITY MANAGEMENT

Beyond detecting current problems, AI enables proactive quality management. Machine learning can predict which data collection activities, time periods, sites, or data sources are most likely to have quality problems, enabling preemptive attention.

Degradation forecasting predicts when quality metrics will fall below acceptable thresholds, enabling intervention before problems become severe. And when quality problems do occur, AI pattern analysis can identify likely root causes, equipment drift, training gaps, protocol ambiguity, and workflow bottlenecks, enabling systemic fixes rather than symptom treatment.

DATA INTEGRITY MONITORING

Consistent with GMLP data integrity principles, AI monitors for unauthorized changes, referential integrity violations, audit trail tampering, data corruption during storage or transfer, and backup validation failures, ensuring that the technical infrastructure that preserves data remains trustworthy.[1] These functions, while less intellectually glamorous than anomaly detection, are foundational: all downstream analysis assumes data integrity, and failures here undermine everything built on top.

SYNTHETIC DATA GENERATION

Synthetic data, artificially generated data that mimics real data characteristics, has evolved from a niche technique to a mainstream tool with significant research applications and an increasingly defined regulatory landscape.

APPLICATIONS

Synthetic data serves various research purposes, each with unique value propositions and validation needs. Privacy protection is the most well-established application: synthetic data allows sharing and analysis without exposing actual individual records, conserving statistical properties while preventing reidentification of real participants.[7] Data augmentation tackles the practical issue of limited real data; when sample sizes are small, synthetic examples can enhance machine learning model performance by expanding training datasets. Addressing underrepresentation is a particularly important use: synthetic data can fill gaps in real datasets by generating examples representing populations that are underrepresented, potentially reducing the algorithmic bias that affects models trained on nonrepresentative samples.[8]

Additional applications include hypothesis exploration (creating synthetic data to test analytical methods with hypothetical scenarios before collecting real data), software testing (verifying data systems and analytical pipelines without using sensitive data), education and training (teaching analysis techniques without accessing protected data), and simulation studies (Monte Carlo simulations and methodological research that require multiple datasets with known properties).

GENERATION APPROACHES

Multiple AI techniques generate synthetic data, each with their own strengths and limitations. Statistical methods, which involve sampling from fitted distributions, are the simplest and most interpretable, maintaining specified marginal distributions and correlations but are limited in capturing complex multivariate relationships. Generative adversarial networks (GANs), featuring a dual-network setup where a generator creates increasingly realistic synthetic data by competing against a discriminator that tries to distinguish synthetic from real data, can model complex data structures but are hard to train and may experience mode collapse (producing data that only covers part of the real data distribution).[9] Variational autoencoders learn compressed representations and generate new examples by sampling from the learned latent space, offering more stable training than GANs with slightly less sharp outputs. Diffusion models, which learn to reverse a noise-adding process, have become powerful generators for both image and tabular clinical data, with recent studies showing they produce superior fidelity and privacy preservation compared to GANs for healthcare applications. Large language models generate synthetic text data (such as clinical notes, survey responses, and narrative records) that closely imitate real data characteristics. Hybrid approaches combining multiple methods address specific needs, such as GANs with differential privacy guarantees, conditional models that produce data matching certain demographic features, or ensemble methods that combine the advantages of several generators.[9]

VALIDATION REQUIREMENTS

Synthetic data is only useful if they are demonstrably fit for purpose, and validation must consider multiple aspects. Utility assessment checks whether analyses on synthetic data produce results similar to those from real data for intended use cases, addressing the core question of whether synthetic data actually works. Privacy assessment determines if synthetic data sufficiently protects individual privacy, using formal guarantees (differential privacy) or empirical reidentification testing.[10] Distributional fidelity assessment evaluates whether synthetic data distributions match real data across marginal distributions, correlations, and higher-order statistical properties relevant to intended analyses. Edge case evaluation investigates whether rare but important cases, which are often the most scientifically interesting, are adequately represented. Temporal dynamics assessment confirms that longitudinal patterns are preserved in synthetic time-series data. Additionally, domain expert review can identify implausible patterns that statistical validation may miss, such as combinations of clinical features that would never cooccur in real patients.

Industry experience indicates that thorough validation should set quantitative benchmarks beforehand, such as requiring fidelity metrics above 85% while avoiding excessive memorization of training data, and these metrics should be reported transparently in any publication or regulatory submission using synthetic data.[11]

THE EVOLVING REGULATORY LANDSCAPE FOR SYNTHETIC DATA

The regulatory approach to synthetic data is quickly taking shape, establishing a framework that researchers need to understand.

The EU AI Act, which took effect in August 2024 with full implementation expected by August 2026, explicitly includes synthetic data in several provisions.[12] Article 10(5)(a) allows the use of synthetic data when real-world data is insufficient for bias detection and correction, showing strong support for synthetic data to promote fairness. Article 50(2) requires AI systems that generate synthetic content (audio, video, text, and images) to label outputs as artificially created, a transparency rule that directly impacts synthetic data in research. Additionally, Article 59(1)(b) considers synthetic data a compliant alternative when anonymized or other nonpersonal data does not meet regulatory standards. These provisions present both opportunities (clear regulatory backing for synthetic data in certain cases) and obligations (labeling, documentation, and validation requirements).

The FDA's January 2025 draft guidance on Considerations for the Use of Artificial Intelligence to Support Regulatory Decision-Making addresses AI-generated data in drug and biological product development, setting expectations for transparency, reproducibility, and validation of AI outputs used in regulatory submissions.[13] While this guidance does not directly specify standards for synthetic data, it outlines the regulatory expectations within which synthetic data use in clinical research will be assessed. EMA guidance specifically focused on synthetic data for data augmentation and differential privacy techniques is anticipated by mid-2026.[12]

NIST's Special Publication 800-226 (2025) clarifies technical requirements for differential privacy claims, including acceptable epsilon ranges, providing concrete benchmarks for the privacy guarantees that synthetic data generators should meet.[14] And the European Data Protection Board's Opinion 28/2024 introduces a three-step legality test for synthetic data under GDPR, listing technical and organizational measures needed to demonstrate model anonymity.[15]

In January 2026, the FDA and EMA jointly issued ten guiding principles for AI in drug development, highlighting data quality, transparency, and validation requirements for synthetic data used in regulatory settings.[16]

ETHICAL CONSIDERATIONS FOR SYNTHETIC DATA

Synthetic data raises ethical concerns that its technical benefits can hide. Transparency is crucial: researchers must clearly state when synthetic data is used, how it was created, and what validation was done. Publications, analyses, and downstream applications should clearly show synthetic data involvement, a requirement supported by the EU AI Act's labeling rules.

Bias propagation is a major concern. Synthetic data derived from biased real data will inherit and possibly amplify those biases. The potential of synthetic data for addressing underrepresentation is genuine but depends on conditions: deliberately adjusting synthetic distributions to fix known biases requires careful scientific backing and transparent reporting to prevent creating artifacts that could be mistaken for real results.[8]

Consent implications are increasingly scrutinized. Using real participant data to train synthetic data generators may not have been considered in original consent forms, raising questions about whether existing consent covers this secondary use. As synthetic data becomes more common, consent language needs to evolve to address it explicitly.

And the potential for misuse, such as using synthetic data to fabricate research results or create misleading datasets, requires that mechanisms for maintaining scientific integrity evolve alongside the technology. Watermarking synthetic data, maintaining provenance records linking synthetic datasets to their creation processes, and developing detection methods for fabricated data are all active areas of development.

DATA GOVERNANCE AND STEWARDSHIP

AI-era data management needs governance frameworks that handle both traditional data stewardship issues and the new challenges AI brings.

GOVERNANCE STRUCTURES

Effective data governance relies on institutional infrastructure: data governance committees with authority over policies, quality standards, access decisions, and compliance monitoring; designated data stewards responsible for specific datasets or domains; clear accountability for data quality, security, privacy, and compliance at each lifecycle stage; comprehensive policies covering collection, storage, quality, access, sharing, retention, and destruction; and compliance mechanisms for monitoring adherence and addressing violations. These structures are not new, but AI enhances their importance by increasing the volume, complexity, and speed of data processing, creating more opportunities for governance failures with wider repercussions.

ACCESS CONTROL AND SECURITY

AI systems that process research data need proper access governance based on data sensitivity. Role-based access controls permissions by function rather than individual. Limiting access to what's needed reduces exposure. Monitoring and logging help identify unusual access patterns. Classifying data by sensitivity allows for appropriate protection. Secure computation environments, including federated approaches that analyze data without centralizing it, enable sensitive data analysis while minimizing exposure risks.

DATA SHARING GOVERNANCE

Research data sharing, which is essential for reproducibility and scientific progress, requires governance that balances openness with protection. Data use agreements that specify permitted uses, security requirements, and compliance obligations create legal frameworks. Deidentification standards aligned with regulatory requirements establish technical standards. Controlled access mechanisms handle requests for sensitive data through review processes and monitoring. And FAIR principles implementation guarantees that shared data is discoverable, accessible, interoperable, and reusable through proper documentation and formats.[4]

LONG-TERM STEWARDSHIP

Research data must outlive the projects that create it, requiring active stewardship modeled on established preservation standards. This includes developing retention policies that balance research value, regulatory requirements, and storage costs; planning for format migration to prevent technical obsolescence[17]; and preserving documentation alongside data over time.

Furthermore, effective stewardship requires formal succession planning to ensure data remains discoverable and usable if the original researchers leave or the host institution can no longer sustain the collection. Such planning is a core requirement of the TRUST Principles (Transparency, Responsibility, User focus, Sustainability, and Technology), which mandate that digital repositories have documented plans for the long-term continuity of data access.[18] Selecting appropriate repositories that adhere to these standards is essential; data that cannot be found, understood, or used is effectively lost, no matter how carefully it was collected.

CAPABILITIES AND LIMITATIONS: THE DATA MANAGEMENT AUDIT

While the Master Matrix in Chapter 1 outlines general AI strengths in Code and Scripting and Information Processing, applying these to data management requires a rigorous set of Integrity Override Triggers. Data management is the foundation of the research enterprise; an undetected AI error at this stage propagates into every subsequent analysis, model, and conclusion. AI excels at the systematic, high-volume tasks of integration and monitoring, but it lacks the Clinical Intuition to distinguish a breakthrough from a typo (Table 13.1).

TABLE 13.1
Data-Specific Override Protocols

Data Management Task	AI Execution (The "Meat")	The Human Override (The Top Bread)
Multisource integration	Harmonizing disparate datasets (EHR, wearables, genomics) into a unified structure	E2B(R3) Compliance Audit: Manually verify that the output meets the April 1, 2026 mandatory standard. Reject legacy "R2" XML files

(*Continued*)

TABLE 13.1 (*Continued*)
Data-Specific Override Protocols

Data Management Task	AI Execution (The "Meat")	The Human Override (The Top Bread)
Synthetic augmentation	Generating "look-alike" datasets to increase power or protect privacy	Diversity/Mode-Collapse Check: Verify the AI hasn't erased rare patient subtypes. Compare synthetic versus real distribution
Automated data cleaning	Identifying and "correcting" missing values or duplicates	QMSR/ISO 13485 Validation: Ensure cleaning logic is documented in a risk-based validation log required by the Feb 2, 2026 transition
Metadata generation	Automatically tagging datasets for searchability and storage	Governance Check: A human data steward must approve the "Consent Scope" tags. AI cannot judge the ethical boundaries of secondary data use

Refer to the Master Matrix in Chapter 1 for foundational failure modes; the table defines the expert-level interventions required for data governance and cleaning.

THE "SANITIZATION" TRAP AND CLINICAL SIGNIFICANCE

A primary limitation in AI-driven data management is the Normalcy Bias. AI models are designed to identify and "smooth out" variance. In a research setting, however, the variance is often the most important data point.

- **The AI Limit**: AI cannot reliably tell the difference between a transcription error and a rare clinical presentation. It treats a "physiologically extreme" value as a statistical error to be corrected.

- **The Human Task**: You must provide the Scientific Context. When the AI flags a value as "out of range," the human investigator must determine if the outlier is an artifact of the collection process or a signal of a novel biological phenomenon. In data management, "clean" is not always "correct."

GOVERNANCE, ETHICS, AND THE "PASSED" 2026 DEADLINES

- **The E2B(R3) Cutoff**: As of the April 1, 2026 deadline, the FDA no longer accepts legacy E2B(R2) formats for safety reporting. AI tools that default to legacy XML structures now trigger immediate rejections at the FDA Electronic Submission Gateway.[19]
- **Informed Consent Scope**: AI can match keywords but cannot perform the Moral Deliberation required to decide if a research goal fits the "spirit" of original consent.
- **Proportionality in Privacy**: AI-driven privacy tools often trade off Utility for Anonymity. Only a human scientist can decide if the "noise" added by the AI has rendered the dataset scientifically useless.

The Override Trigger: If the AI suggests a data-cleaning step that removes more than [X]% of your raw outliers or fails to provide a 21 CFR Part 11-compliant audit trail, you must trigger a Data Integrity Bypass. You are the final steward of the evidence; the AI is merely the processor of the bits.

THE SKEPTIC'S CORNER

- **Target Task**: Synthetic data and Regulatory Compliance.
- **Adversarial Prompt**: "This synthetic dataset claims 90% fidelity. Identify if it has experienced 'Mode Collapse' regarding our rare disease cohort. Furthermore, verify if the metadata meets the April 1, 2026 E2B(R3) requirements for electronic transmission to the FDA."

ETHICAL CONSIDERATIONS

AI in data collection and management raises ethical issues across multiple dimensions that demand proactive attention instead of reactive responses.

PRIVACY AND CONFIDENTIALITY

The privacy risks introduced in Chapter 9 take specific forms in data management. AI can enable reidentification of supposedly deidentified data through linking datasets, inferring from patterns, or exploiting data sparsity, especially as more datasets become accessible for cross-referencing. Its capacity to extract information from data may conflict with data minimization principles emphasized by privacy regulations. Continuous AI monitoring of data quality could lead to inappropriate surveillance of researchers or participants if not properly managed. Additionally, the secondary use of AI-extracted information might surpass the scope of the original consent, requiring careful review of what the consent covers and what needs additional authorization.

BIAS AND EQUITY

The bias and equity concerns discussed in Chapter 9 are particularly structural in data management. AI systems trained on historically biased data will continue existing biases, consistently underrepresenting populations that are already marginalized.[8] AI quality assessments may identify data from certain groups as problematic, for example, labeling culturally specific response patterns as "anomalies," which can introduce bias into the quality assurance process itself. Advanced AI data systems available only to well-funded institutions create capability gaps, giving advantages to some researchers while disadvantaging others. Additionally, while synthetic data shows promise for reducing underrepresentation, its effectiveness depends on careful generation and validation; poorly created synthetic data may give a false impression of representation without substantive accuracy.

TRANSPARENCY AND ACCOUNTABILITY

The transparency and accountability principles discussed in Chapter 9 apply directly to data processing: publications should specify which AI systems processed their data and how; AI quality decisions should be auditable, with clear records of what was flagged, excluded, and corrected; and sufficient documentation should enable reproduction of all AI data-processing steps.

INFORMED CONSENT

Consent considerations for AI data management involve transparency about when AI will be involved in collecting or processing participant data, careful attention to consent for synthetic data generation (which original consent may not have covered), disclosure of ongoing learning if AI systems adapt over time based on participant data, and notification when AI influences decisions affecting participants using their data. As AI becomes more integrated into research data systems, consent language must be updated to clearly address these specific uses, rather than relying on broad authorizations that participants might not have fully understood to include AI processing.

PRACTICAL IMPLEMENTATION

Organizations adopting AI data management should view it as a step-by-step process rather than a complete overhaul.

PHASED IMPLEMENTATION

Following the phased implementation approach described in Chapter 1, data management implementation begins with assessment, inventorying current processes, applying the NIST Map function to understand data contexts and risks, and developing governance frameworks. Pilot deployment on limited scope with extensive human oversight builds organizational experience before expanded deployment extends successful approaches across the institution.

TECHNOLOGY AND WORKFORCE CONSIDERATIONS

Technology selection should focus on integration with existing research infrastructure and on open standards to prevent lock-in, as discussed in more detail in Chapter 12. Workforce development is just as important: researchers need training not only in AI data tools but also on their limitations and quality oversight requirements, and institutions need specialized data science expertise to support increasingly complex data pipelines.

QUALITY MANAGEMENT INTEGRATION

AI data tools must integrate with quality management systems through established performance metrics (accuracy, completeness, timeliness, and efficiency), validation protocols for deployment and regular reassessment, deviation management processes for addressing AI failures, continuous improvement driven by quality data, and audit readiness with detailed documentation. These quality management functions, aligned with NIST's Manage function, ensure that AI data tools remain trustworthy as data environments, study requirements, and AI systems evolve over time.[3]

LOOKING FORWARD

AI in data management continues to evolve rapidly across various areas. Multimodal AI, which seamlessly combines text, images, audio, video, and sensor data, will allow for richer data collection and more advanced quality assessment than what modality-specific tools can offer. Foundation models tailored for research data will deliver powerful capabilities with less need for domain-specific training. Edge computing will enable AI processing directly at data collection points, eliminating centralized data transfer and enhancing privacy and efficiency. Federated learning will enable model training across multiple distributed datasets without centralizing data, allowing learning from sensitive information while maintaining privacy.

Standards are evolving simultaneously. Guidance on synthetic data from regulators (FDA, EMA, and MHRA) is expected to clarify validation requirements and suitable applications by 2026–2027. FAIR[2] and similar AI-readiness standards for data management will make research datasets easier to process automatically while keeping the documentation needed for human interpretation.[5] International efforts to harmonize standards aim for consistency in AI research data management across different jurisdictions, which is important as research becomes more global and data crosses regulatory borders.

The trajectory is clear: AI will become deeply integrated into research data infrastructure, managing volume, velocity, and complexity that manual methods cannot handle. The challenge is to ensure this integration promotes scientific quality, safeguards participant privacy, fosters equity, and upholds the transparency essential for scientific accountability. This challenge mainly involves governance and human judgment, supported by technology but not reducible to it.

The next chapter explores how AI can assist with data analysis and interpretation, building on the quality data foundations discussed here.

KEY TAKEAWAYS

- AI transforms data collection through automated capture, adaptive sampling, real-time quality monitoring, and multimodal integration, but each capability introduces error modes that require human oversight.
- GMLP principles prioritize data quality as fundamental, highlighting the importance of representative data, suitable reference standards, and real-world performance monitoring.
- FUTURE-AI traceability demands comprehensive documentation, provenance tracking, version control, and audit trails. AI makes this feasible by automatically maintaining records during data operations.
- The NIST AI RMF Map function helps researchers understand data contexts, identify stakeholders, and assess data-related risks before deploying AI tools.

- FAIR and $FAIR^2$ principles ensure data benefits both human researchers and AI systems through machine-readable metadata, standardized formats, and clear documentation.
- Data quality assurance moves from periodic manual checks to continuous AI monitoring, identifying issues at the collection stage instead of after contamination.
- Synthetic data supports privacy, enhances data augmentation, and tackles underrepresentation, while an evolving regulatory landscape (EU AI Act, FDA, and NIST) sets validation requirements and allowed uses.
- Governance structures, access controls, sharing frameworks, and long-term stewardship planning are essential infrastructure for data management in the AI era.
- Human judgment remains essential for identifying errors versus outliers, interpreting data within context, making governance decisions, and ensuring AI data tools uphold scientific integrity.

QUESTIONS FOR REFLECTION

1. How can AI-assisted data collection enhance data quality in your research while ensuring proper human oversight, and what error modes should you monitor?
2. What documentation and provenance tracking would FUTURE-AI traceability principles require for your research data, and how could AI assist in maintaining these records without imposing an unsustainable documentation burden?
3. How could synthetic data benefit your research, whether for privacy, augmentation, or equity, and what validation is necessary to confirm it's suitable for its intended purpose?
4. What data-related risks would the NIST Map function identify in your research, and how should data collection and management proactively address these risks?

5. How is your institution preparing for the changing regulatory environment regarding synthetic data and AI-processed research data, including EU AI Act requirements and new FDA guidance?
6. How should your institution balance AI efficiency in data management with the need for human judgment in quality decisions, and what governance structures would support maintaining that balance?

NOTES

1. International Medical Device Regulators Forum. (2025). Good machine learning practice for medical device development: Guiding principles. IMDRF/AIML WG/N88 FINAL:2025. https://www.fda.gov/medical-devices/software-medical-device-samd/good-machine-learning-practice-medical-device-development-guiding-principles. Note: Ten guiding principles finalized by IMDRF in January 2025, building on the original 2021 joint statement by the FDA, Health Canada, and UK MHRA with broader international endorsement and updates including expanded considerations for generative AI, enhanced lifecycle monitoring, and updated data representation requirements. Principles 2 (robust software engineering), 3 (representative datasets), 5 (fit-for-purpose reference standards), and 10 (postdeployment monitoring) are particularly relevant to research data management, establishing that data quality is foundational to trustworthy AI.
2. Lekadir, K., et al. (2025). FUTURE-AI: International consensus guideline for trustworthy and deployable artificial intelligence in healthcare. *BMJ*, 388, e081554. https://doi.org/10.1136/bmj-2024-081554. Note: International consensus identifying six core principles, Fairness, Universality, Traceability, Usability, Robustness, and Explainability, for trustworthy AI in healthcare. The traceability principle provides the most comprehensive framework for data provenance, documentation, and version control requirements in AI-enabled research.
3. National Institute of Standards and Technology. (2023). Artificial intelligence risk management framework (AI RMF 1.0). NIST AI 100-1. https://www.nist.gov/itl/ai-risk-management-framework. Note: The four-function framework (Govern, Map, Measure, and Manage) applied to data management: the Map function guides

understanding of data contexts, stakeholders, and risks; the Measure function tracks quality metrics; and the Manage function directs mitigation and improvement.

4. Wilkinson, M. D., et al. (2016). The FAIR guiding principles for scientific data management and stewardship. *Scientific Data*, 3, 160018. https://doi.org/10.1038/sdata.2016.18. Note: The foundational articulation of Findable, Accessible, Interoperable, and Reusable principles for scientific data, now the standard framework for data stewardship globally. The 15 guiding principles (F1-F4, A1-A2, I1-I3, R1-R1.3) provide measurable, implementable standards.
5. Frontiers. (2025, March 3). Reimagining FAIR for an AI world: Frontiers introduces FAIR^2 data management. https://www.frontiersin.org/news/2025/03/03/reimagining-fair-for-an-ai-world-frontiers-introduces-fair-data-management. Note: FAIR^2 (FAIR Squared) extends the original FAIR principles by adding AI-readiness requirements, integrating data with provenance, methodology, and detailed data dictionaries to create context-rich, machine-actionable datasets. Compatible with MLCommons Croissant AI-ready format and major AI frameworks (TensorFlow, JAX, PyTorch). Represents the convergence of open science data principles and AI infrastructure requirements.
6. FDA 2026. Quality management system regulation (QMSR). https://www.fda.gov/medical-devices/postmarket-requirements-devices/quality-management-system-regulation-qmsr
7. El Emam, K., Mosquera, L., & Hoptroff, R. (2020). *Practical Synthetic Data Generation: Balancing Privacy and the Broad Availability of Data*. O'Reilly Media. Note: The most comprehensive practical guide to synthetic data generation, covering privacy-utility tradeoffs, generation techniques, evaluation methods, and implementation strategies. Particularly valuable for researchers new to synthetic data who need both conceptual understanding and practical guidance.
8. Chen, R. J., Lu, M. Y., Chen, T. Y., Williamson, D. F. K., & Mahmood, F. (2021). Synthetic data in machine learning for medicine and healthcare. *Nature Biomedical Engineering*, 5(6), 493–497. https://doi.org/10.1038/s41551-021-00751-8. Note: Examines both the promise and vulnerabilities of synthetic data in healthcare AI, including bias propagation risks when synthetic data inherits biases from training data, the potential for addressing underrepresentation, and the challenges of validation and quality assurance.

9. Goodfellow, I., Pouget-Abadie, J., Mirza, M., Xu, B., Warde-Farley, D., Ozair, S., Courville, A., & Bengio, Y. (2014). Generative adversarial nets. *Advances in Neural Information Processing Systems*, 27, 2672–2680. Note: The seminal paper introducing the GAN architecture, a generator network trained adversarially against a discriminator, that has become a foundational technique for synthetic data generation across domains.
10. Jordon, J., et al. (2022). Synthetic data, what, why and how? *arXiv preprint* arXiv:2205.03257. https://arxiv.org/abs/2205.03257. Note: Comprehensive overview of synthetic data technologies covering generation methods, evaluation frameworks (utility, fidelity, privacy), privacy-preserving approaches including differential privacy, applications for fairness and data augmentation, and a survey of generative model architectures.
11. IntuitionLabs. (2025, revised February 2026). Synthetic data in pharma: A guide to acceptance criteria. https://intuitionlabs.ai/articles/synthetic-data-pharma-acceptance-criteria. Note: Comprehensive analysis of regulatory momentum around synthetic data in pharmaceutical contexts, documenting FDA/EMA joint principles for AI in drug development, MHRA draft guidelines on external control arms (May 2025), and practical acceptance criteria (fidelity ≥85%, privacy validation, and no excessive memorization) that researchers can apply to validate synthetic data for regulatory and scientific purposes.
12. European Parliament and Council of the European Union. (2024). Regulation (EU) 2024/1689 laying down harmonised rules on artificial intelligence (AI Act). *Official Journal of the European Union*. https://artificialintelligenceact.eu. Note: Articles 10(5)(a), 50(2), and 59(1)(b) explicitly address synthetic data, permitting its use for bias detection when real data are insufficient, requiring labeling of AI-generated synthetic content, and recognizing synthetic data as a compliant alternative to anonymized data when the latter is insufficient. Full applicability August 2, 2026.
13. U.S. Food and Drug Administration. (2025). Considerations for the use of artificial intelligence to support regulatory decision-making for drug and biological products, draft guidance. https://www.fda.gov/regulatory-information/search-fda-guidance-documents/considerations-use-artificial-intelligence-support-regulatory-decision-making-drug-and-biological. Note: Establishes expectations for transparency, reproducibility, and validation of AI-generated outputs used in regulatory submissions for drugs and biologics. While not prescribing synthetic data standards directly, it frames the regulatory context within which AI-generated and AI-processed research data will be evaluated.

14. Near, J. P., Darais, D., Lefkovitz, N., & Howarth, G. S. (2025). Guidelines for evaluating differential privacy guarantees. (National Institute of Standards and Technology, Gaithersburg, MD), NIST Special Publication (SP) NIST SP 800-226. NIST. SP.800-226.pdf
15. European Data Protection Board (EDPB). (2024). Opinion 28/2024 on certain data protection aspects related to the processing of personal data in the context of AI models. Adopted on 17 December 2024. Retrieved from: edpb_opinion_202428_ai-models_en.pdf
16. EMA (Jan 2026). Guiding principles of good AI practice in drug development. https://www.ema.europa.eu/en/documents/other/guiding-principles-good-ai-practice-drug-development_en.pdf
17. ISO 14721:2012. Space data and information transfer systems, Open archival information system (OAIS), Reference model. International Organization for Standardization. Note: This is the primary international standard that defines the requirement for "Digital Migration."
18. Lin, D., et al. (2020). The TRUST Principles for digital repositories. *Scientific Data*, 7(1), 144. https://doi.org/10.1038/s41597-020-0486-7
19. FDA Adverse Event Reporting System (FAERS). Electronic submissions – E2B(R3) standards. https://www.fda.gov/drugs/fda-adverse-event-monitoring-system-aems/fda-adverse-event-reporting-system-faers-electronic-submissions-e2br3-standards, accessed July 16, 2026.

14 Data Analysis and Interpretation

THE CHALLENGE OF MODERN RESEARCH DATA ANALYSIS

The data landscape researchers face today is fundamentally different from what traditional statistical methods were built to handle. Recognizing why AI analysis has become necessary instead of just trendy requires clearly understanding these differences.

High dimensionality is likely the most significant change. Genomic research often produces datasets with millions of variables (such as single nucleotide polymorphisms [SNPs], gene expression levels, and epigenetic markers) for hundreds or thousands of participants, creating a variable-to-observation ratio that breaks the assumptions of traditional regression methods. Neuroimaging yields hundreds of thousands of voxel measurements per scan. Natural language processing (NLP) treats each word or token as a possible variable. In these cases, traditional techniques either cannot be used or require such extensive dimension reduction that critical signals might be lost before analysis even starts. Machine learning (ML) methods, built for high-dimensional data, find meaningful patterns where standard techniques falter.

Complex relationships increase the difficulty of understanding dimensionality. Real-world phenomena involve nonlinear effects, interactions, conditional dependencies, and threshold behaviors that linear models cannot capture. A drug's effect may depend on a patient's genetic profile, which interacts with comorbidities that vary by age and sex, an intricate web of relationships too complex for manually specified interaction terms but well suited for flexible ML methods. The risk, of course, is that this flexibility also allows models to "discover" spurious patterns reflecting noise rather than

DOI 10.1201/9781003782995-19

true signals, highlighting the tension between modeling capacity and scientific rigor that permeates this entire chapter.

Data heterogeneity introduces another layer. Research increasingly merges structured numerical data with medical images, clinical text, audio recordings, video, sensor streams, and social media data. AI offers unified frameworks for analyzing various modalities and uncovering cross-modal relationships, enabling predictions of clinical outcomes from combined imaging, genomic, and clinical data, something that traditional modality-specific methods cannot do.

Scale, missing data, streaming data, and reproducibility demands all contribute to an analytical environment where AI is not a luxury but a necessity for many research programs. The challenge is deploying these powerful tools with the rigor that scientific conclusions require, validation, interpretation, robustness, and transparency, rather than treating AI as a black box that transforms data into discoveries.

FOUNDATIONAL FRAMEWORKS FOR AI ANALYSIS

Three frameworks offer structured guidance for responsible AI use in research analytics. They focus on different yet complementary aspects of analytical rigor.

FUTURE-AI ROBUSTNESS

While Chapter 13 examined these frameworks through the lens of data quality and traceability, here I focus on their implications for analytical rigor and validation. The FUTURE-AI international consensus guideline identifies robustness as one of six core principles for trustworthy AI in healthcare, with direct application to research analytics.[1] Robustness in this context means several things at once. Reliable performance under different conditions: analyses that yield consistent results across various data samples, time periods, and contexts lay the foundation for scientific conclusions, while analyses that only work under narrow conditions do not. Resistance to perturbations: small changes in input data or parameters should cause only small changes in output, not drastically different conclusions. Graceful degradation: when conditions deviate from expectations (such as imperfect data quality or partially violated assumptions), robust systems produce degraded but still meaningful results rather than failing catastrophically. And temporal stability: models trained on historical data should perform reliably on future data, and this stability should be monitored rather than assumed.

For research analytics, robustness means a clear requirement: analyses must produce reliable, reproducible results across reasonable variations in data and methods. An "insight" that appears only with one specific preprocessing pipeline, one model specification, and one particular data split is not a scientific finding; it is an artifact.

GOOD MACHINE LEARNING PRACTICE (GMLP) VALIDATION REQUIREMENTS

The GMLP guiding principles establish validation standards that broadly apply to AI analysis in research.[2] Several principles are especially important. Independent validation, which involves testing on data separate from the training data, avoids the problem of circular reasoning by not evaluating a model on the same data used to develop it. Using validation data that accurately reflects the populations and conditions where the analyses will be applied helps prevent the common issue of validating models on convenient but unrepresentative samples. Correct reference standards, such as ground truth or gold-standard measurements of sufficient quality, ensure validation measures provide meaningful results. Additionally, ongoing validation, which involves monitoring performance over time instead of treating validation as a one-time event, helps detect degradation that naturally occurs as conditions change.

NIST AI RMF MEASURE FUNCTION

The NIST AI Risk Management Framework's Measure function offers structured approaches to assessing AI system performance that go beyond basic accuracy metrics.[3] It highlights quantitative metrics suitable for the analytical task (accuracy, precision, recall, calibration, and domain-specific measures), qualitative evaluation of trustworthiness traits (transparency, explainability, and fairness) that numbers alone cannot fully capture, contextual analysis considering how the results will be used and the potential consequences of errors, uncertainty quantification that reflects the reliability of outcomes, and benchmarking against existing methods, human experts, or established baselines. For research analytics, the Measure function's focus on comprehensive, context-aware evaluation counteracts the tendency to reduce model assessment to a single performance figure.

AI FOR EXPLORATORY DATA ANALYSIS

Before conducting formal hypothesis testing, researchers need to understand their data, including its structure, quality, patterns, and potential issues. AI significantly improves this exploratory phase.

AUTOMATED PROFILING AND PATTERN DISCOVERY

AI can systematically analyze datasets in ways that would take human analysts weeks of manual work. Automated distribution analysis detects skewness, multimodality, outliers, and other features needing attention across all variables at once. Relationship detection, using ML to find correlations, nonlinear associations, and conditional dependencies, provides an initial understanding of data structure that guides both quality assessment and analysis planning. Missing data characterization helps determine whether missingness is random, systematic, or structured, an important distinction for selecting proper handling methods. Additionally, anomaly detection flags unusual observations, unexpected patterns, or quality issues that require investigation before formal analysis.

DIMENSIONALITY REDUCTION AND VISUALIZATION

When datasets contain thousands of variables, understanding their structure requires reducing dimensionality to something human cognition can process. Principal component analysis and its variants identify major axes of variation. Manifold learning techniques, t-SNE, UMAP,[4] and autoencoders, discover low-dimensional structures underlying high-dimensional data, enabling visualization that reveals clusters, gradients, and outliers invisible in raw high-dimensional space. Unsupervised clustering identifies natural groupings, patient subgroups, behavioral clusters, and experimental conditions with similar profiles, which suggest hypotheses for formal testing.

The exploratory power of these tools is real, but so are the risks. Dimensionality reduction leads to information loss; different techniques can create various visualizations of the same data; and algorithmically identified clusters may not match meaningful biological or behavioral groups. Exploratory findings should lead to hypotheses, not final conclusions, a point that modern visualization tools' ease and visual appeal can dangerously obscure.

STATISTICAL ANALYSIS AND HYPOTHESIS TESTING

AI improves traditional statistical analysis by allowing researchers to ask a broader range of questions while preserving, when used correctly, the scientific rigor needed for valid conclusions.

ENHANCED STATISTICAL METHODS

ML offers robust estimators that better tolerate outliers, model misspecification, and other violations of traditional assumptions than conventional methods. Regularization techniques, including least absolute shrinkage and selection operator (LASSO or L1 regularization),[5] ridge regression, and elastic net, enable estimation when variables outnumber observations, while simultaneously selecting important predictors and preventing overfitting. The LASSO, introduced by Tibshirani in 1996, remains one of the most popular tools in high-dimensional statistics because it strikes a balance between flexibility and simplicity: by penalizing the sum of absolute coefficient values, it sets many coefficients exactly to zero, resulting in sparse, interpretable models.

Bayesian methods, supported by modern computational tools like Markov chain Monte Carlo[6] and variational inference,[7] allow for principled uncertainty quantification and the seamless integration of prior knowledge.[8] These are especially useful in research areas where prior information is available but sample sizes are small. Semiparametric and nonparametric methods provide flexible modeling options without relying on strict distributional assumptions. Additionally, AI-enhanced causal inference techniques, such as propensity score matching, doubly robust estimation, instrumental variable approaches, and difference-in-differences with ML, strengthen causal conclusions from observational data, although they are still subject to untestable assumptions inherent in observational causal inference.

MULTIPLE TESTING AND FALSE DISCOVERY CONTROL

High-dimensional analysis introduces a massive multiple testing problem. Genome-wide association studies examine millions of genetic variants; neuroimaging analyses evaluate hundreds of thousands of voxels; text mining explores thousands of potential associations. Without proper correction, the risk of false positive "discoveries" outweighs genuine findings.

Modern false discovery rate (FDR) methods, pioneered by the Benjamini–Hochberg procedure[9] and the *q*-value approach,[10] control the expected proportion of false positives among reported findings, allowing for large-scale testing while keeping false discoveries within acceptable limits. In the context of AI-driven discovery, researchers should employ more advanced adaptive techniques:

- **Empirical Bayes Adaptive Shrinkage**: Methods like ashr[11] provide more accurate FDR control by using the entire dataset to "shrink" effect estimates, which is particularly effective when dealing with many small, noisy clinical signals.
- **The Knockoff Filter**: For high-dimensional variable selection where p-values are difficult to calculate, the Knockoff filter[12] provides a robust framework by creating "synthetic controls" for every variable to ensure the FDR is strictly controlled.

- **Weighted FDR**: When biological plausibility is known, weighted FDR procedures[13] allow researchers to integrate prior knowledge, such as known metabolic pathways or genetic clusters, into the discovery threshold.

Selective inference methods tackle the more subtle issue of testing hypotheses suggested by the same data used to generate them, a common practice in exploratory-then-confirmatory analysis that can invalidate standard inference if not properly addressed. Resampling methods, including the bootstrap, permutation tests, and cross-validation, provide a framework for valid inference that does not rely on rigid distributional assumptions (e.g., normality), broadening the range of situations where reliable conclusions can be made from complex biomedical data.[14]

POWER AND SAMPLE SIZE

AI enhances study planning through simulation-based power analysis that manages designs too complex for analytical formulas, adaptive designs that adjust procedures based on growing data while maintaining statistical validity, and optimal allocation methods that distribute samples across conditions or sites to maximize power within constraints. These planning tools assist researchers in avoiding both underpowered studies that waste resources and overpowered studies that detect trivially small effects.

PREDICTIVE MODELING AND ML

Predictive modeling, which uses data to forecast outcomes for new observations, is one of the most developed AI applications in research, with established methodological frameworks and validation standards.

MODEL DEVELOPMENT

Building predictive models that generalize beyond training data requires a disciplined methodology. Algorithm selection should be guided by problem characteristics rather than trends: linear models for interpretable prediction with moderate complexity; tree-based methods (random forests, gradient boosting) for handling interactions and mixed variable types; neural networks for complex patterns in large datasets; and ensemble methods for robustness that no single algorithm can match. Feature engineering, domain-informed transformations, interaction terms, and temporal aggregations often improve performance more than algorithm sophistication; this serves as a reminder that domain knowledge remains the most valuable analytical resource. Hyperparameter optimization (grid search, random search, and Bayesian optimization) identifies configurations that generalize well rather than simply memorizing training data. Additionally, training procedures like early stopping, learning rate schedules, and data augmentation help prevent overfitting, which is the central challenge of predictive modeling.

VALIDATION STRATEGIES

Rigorous validation distinguishes a useful model from a misleading one, and GMLP requirements offer the framework.[2] K-fold cross-validation, which involves repeatedly training on subsets and validating on held-out data, provides unbiased estimates of performance for internal validation.

Temporal and Spatial Validation: Temporal validation, where training occurs on earlier data and validation on later data, is crucial for time-series applications because standard cross-validation can violate temporal order and produce overly optimistic estimates. External validation on independent datasets from different institutions, populations, or time periods provides the strongest evidence of generalizability and is increasingly required for the publication of prediction models.

Subgroup and Calibration Assessment: Subgroup validation evaluates performance across demographic groups, disease subtypes, and study conditions, identifying populations where models perform differently. Furthermore, calibration assessment, measuring how well predicted probabilities match observed frequencies, determines whether predictions can be trusted for clinical decision-making. Researchers must move beyond simple discrimination metrics area under the receiver operating characteristics curve (AUC/ROC) to ensure that the model's predicted risk corresponds to the actual incidence of the event.[15]

HANDLING OVERFITTING

Overfitting, which occurs when models perform exceptionally well on training data but poorly on other data, is the most common failure mode in predictive modeling. Regularization methods like L1, L2, or elastic net penalties help prevent overfitting by discouraging unnecessary complexity. Cross-validation for model selection helps avoid the mistake of choosing models based solely on training performance. Early stopping terminates iterative training before models memorize noise. Dropout and noise injection during neural network training reduce reliance on specific features. Ensemble methods combine multiple models to average out individual quirks. Sometimes, the best approach is to select a simpler model, especially when data is limited, as a well-specified linear model can often generalize better than a deep neural network despite having lower training accuracy.

DEEP LEARNING APPLICATIONS

Deep learning broadens AI's ability to analyze data types that traditional methods can't handle directly.

IMAGE ANALYSIS

Computer vision has achieved impressive results in research settings. Esteva and colleagues showed in 2017 that a deep convolutional neural network trained on about 130,000 skin lesion images could classify skin cancer at the same level as board-certified dermatologists.[16] Since then, deep learning has been used in medical imaging (radiology, pathology, and ophthalmology), microscopy (cell counting, structure identification, and morphological measurement), remote sensing (land use classification, environmental monitoring, and species identification), and behavioral research (action detection, movement tracking, and expression recognition).

NLP

NLP enables research on text data at an unprecedented scale. Information extraction systems pull structured data (entities, relationships, and events) from unstructured clinical notes, scientific literature, and historical documents. Text classification sorts documents by topic, sentiment, or other research-relevant factors. Semantic analysis evaluates meaning, identifies themes, quantifies linguistic features, and detects stance.

At the scale of scientific literature itself, AI processes thousands of papers to identify trends, synthesize findings, discover connections, and generate hypotheses that human reviewers could not accomplish on such a scale.[17] This capability is particularly vital in fields where the publication volume has moved beyond the capacity for manual human synthesis.

Large language models have significantly expanded these NLP capabilities, enabling qualitative data coding (such as assisting with interview transcripts and observational notes), complex literature synthesis, and even automated hypothesis generation. However, the use of these models in formal research requires a higher level of transparency than traditional text mining. The TRIPOD-LLM reporting guideline, published in January 2025 in *Nature Medicine*, now provides the mandatory framework for transparent reporting of studies that use large language models for prediction, ensuring that the scale of discovery is matched by the rigor of scientific documentation.[18]

MULTIMODAL ANALYSIS

Perhaps the most powerful analytical capability AI provides is integrating information across modalities. Cross-modal prediction, predicting imaging findings from clinical text, outcomes from combined clinical and genomic data, and behavioral patterns from sensor and survey data, exploits complementary information that single-modality analysis cannot capture.

INTERPRETABILITY AND EXPLAINABILITY

Understanding what AI analyses reveal is not just desirable for scientific credibility, it is crucial for scientific validity. A prediction model that accurately forecasts outcomes but offers no insight into mechanisms has limited scientific value.

INHERENTLY INTERPRETABLE MODELS

Some model classes are inherently interpretable: linear models with coefficients that show variable effects, decision trees with clear rule structures, and generalized additive models. The common belief that interpretable models must sacrifice predictive performance is often incorrect; in many cases, simpler models perform nearly as well as more complex ones, making interpretability almost costless.

POST HOC EXPLANATION METHODS

When complex models are necessary, post hoc explanation methods like SHapley Additive exPlanations (SHAP) values[19] quantify each feature's contribution to predictions. However, explanations themselves need validation. Faithfulness assessment checks if explanations truly reflect model behavior. Concept-based explanations describe model behavior using human-understandable concepts rather than raw features.[20]

CAUSAL INFERENCE

Moving beyond prediction to understanding, from "what will happen" to "why does it happen," is where AI faces both its greatest analytical opportunities and its most fundamental limitations.

CAUSAL DISCOVERY AND EFFECT ESTIMATION

Algorithms for discovering causal structures from observational data are among the most ambitious applications of AI in research. Constraint-based methods like PC and FCI identify causal relationships based on patterns of conditional independence.[21] Causal effect estimation uses ML to calculate propensity scores, allowing for matching or weighting that simulates randomization.

CAUSAL VALIDITY

Causal inference from observational data relies on assumptions such as no unmeasured confounding and positivity, which are fundamentally untestable. Sensitivity analyses can evaluate how robust conclusions are to potential confounding, but they cannot confirm its absence.

ROBUSTNESS AND RELIABILITY

In line with FUTURE-AI robustness principles, AI analyses must show reliability across reasonable variations in data and methods before their findings can be accepted as scientific conclusions.[1]

ASSESSING ROBUSTNESS

Sensitivity analysis, which involves varying analytical choices such as model specifications and variable definitions, shows how results depend on particular choices. External replication using independent datasets offers the strongest evidence for validity. Additionally, adversarial testing, challenging models with deliberately difficult or out-of-distribution inputs, reveals vulnerabilities that standard evaluations might miss.

SOURCES OF FRAGILITY

Understanding what makes analyses fragile helps in mitigation. Data Leakage is a primary source of fragility; if an AI is trained on a patient's records but tested on a future record from the same patient, the model is "cheating" by using future knowledge to predict the present.[22]

UNCERTAINTY QUANTIFICATION

A valid analysis requires not only point estimates but also an honest characterization of the uncertainty. Conformal prediction, a distribution-free framework providing prediction intervals with guaranteed coverage under minimal assumptions, has emerged as a particularly valuable tool for AI applications.[23]

REPORTING STANDARDS

The transparency needed for scientific reproducibility has been formalized in reporting guidelines.

TRIPOD+AI AND TRIPOD-LLM

The TRIPOD statement was updated in April 2024 as TRIPOD+AI, a 27-item checklist for reporting prediction model studies using ML.[24] For studies using large language models, the TRIPOD-LLM reporting guideline was published in *Nature Medicine* in January 2025.[18] As of early 2026, adherence to these standards is mandatory for high-impact publication.

CAPABILITIES AND LIMITATIONS: THE ANALYTICAL AUDIT

While the Master Matrix in Chapter 1 outlines general AI strengths in Pattern Recognition and Code and Scripting, applying these to formal data analysis requires this book's most rigorous Methodological Override Protocols. AI enables the analysis of high-dimensional, multimodal data at scales previously impossible, but its "flexibility" is a double-edged sword. Without expert human intervention, AI will "discover" patterns in pure noise, leading to the Overfitting and Spurious Discoveries that fuel the reproducibility crisis (Table 14.1).

TABLE 14.1
Analysis-Specific Override Protocols

Analytical Task	AI Execution (The "Meat")	The Human Override (The Top Bread)
Exploratory discovery	Identifying clusters and nonlinear correlations in high-dimensional datasets	**Plausibility Check:** Humans must verify if an AI-identified "cluster" matches a known biological subgroup or is an artifact of the collection site
Predictive modeling	Training complex models (random forests, CNNs) to forecast clinical outcomes	**Calibration and Robustness Audit:** Trigger a manual **Sensitivity Analysis**. Verify that the predicted probabilities match real-world frequencies (Calibration) rather than just ranking patients (Discrimination)
Causal inference	Using algorithms to suggest "Why" a phenomenon happens from observational data	**Confounder Stress Test:** A "hostile statistician" review to identify unmeasured variables (e.g., socioeconomic factors) that the AI cannot "see"
Unstructured extraction	Using NLP or Computer Vision to quantify patterns in text, images, or audio	**Faithfulness Audit:** Manually verify a 5% randomized sample of AI-extracted "features" against the raw source (e.g., the original pathology slide)
Data partitioning	Randomly splitting data into training and testing sets	**Leakage Mitigation:** Mandatory Patient-Level Splitting. Ensure no patient exists in both sets and perform Temporal Partitioning to ensure the "future" is not used to predict the "past"

Refer to the Master Matrix in Chapter 1 for foundational failure modes; the table defines the expert-level interventions required for valid scientific interpretation.

THE "DIMENSIONALITY TRAP" AND SPURIOUS LOGIC

A primary limitation in AI analysis is Overparameterization. When variables (like SNPs or voxels) outnumber observations, AI can "perfectly" map the training data without learning anything about the underlying science.

- **The AI Limit**: AI optimizes for accuracy, not truth. It will use "shortcut features," such as the hospital's specific imaging font or the timestamp of a scan, to make a prediction if those features correlate with the outcome in the training set.
- **The Human Task**: You must provide the Methodological Guardrails. Use the GMLP principles to mandate Independent Validation on a representative dataset. If the model fails when moved to a new clinic, the AI has "memorized" the hospital's specific noise rather than the disease signal.

INTERPRETABILITY VERSUS "THE BLACK BOX"

In 2026, scientific validity depends on Explainability. A model that predicts a 95% survival rate but cannot explain "why" has limited utility for a physician or a participant.

- **Validating the Explanation**: As established in the TRIPOD+AI (2024) and TRIPOD-LLM (2025) guidelines, an AI-generated "explanation" (like a SHAP value) is just an approximation.[17,18,21] It requires a human Clinical Sanity Check to ensure the explanation aligns with established domain knowledge.
- **The "Black Swan" of Robustness**: As noted in the FUTURE-AI framework, an analysis must be robust against "perturbations."[1] If a small change in your data (e.g., removing two outliers) results in a drastically different AI conclusion, the analysis is fragile and must be overridden.

The Override Trigger: Shadow Coding. To ensure analytical integrity, researchers should implement "Shadow Coding" (Independent Redundancy). For any primary outcome, a human statistician should manually reverify the AI's core logic or write a parallel script in a different language (e.g., R versus Python) to confirm the results. If the AI-generated analysis suggests a causal link that fails this independent redundancy check, you must trigger an Analytical Bypass. You are the final arbiter of the scientific conclusion; the AI is merely the processor of the probabilities.

THE SKEPTIC'S CORNER

- **Target Task**: Predictive modeling and causal inference.
- **Adversarial Prompt**: "This causal model suggests that [Variable X] leads to [Outcome Y]. Now, act as a hostile statistician and identify five 'unmeasured confounders' that could explain this correlation without any direct causal link between X and Y. Furthermore, generate a calibration plot to prove that your 90% accuracy isn't just an artifact of a biased training set."

ETHICAL CONSIDERATIONS

AI analysis raises ethical issues that extend beyond methodological rigor to encompass fairness, transparency, privacy, and societal impact.

ALGORITHMIC BIAS

The bias issues discussed in this book, such as training data underrepresentation, different performance across groups, and the need for fairness-aware methods and diverse teams, manifest in specific ways in analysis. Interpretation bias, where findings are viewed through assumptions about which populations are important, affects which outcomes are prioritized and which harms are acknowledged. Publication practices deserve particular attention: if AI-discovered findings are selectively published based on their direction or statistical significance, the scientific literature becomes systematically misleading, a problem made worse by AI's ability to test thousands of hypotheses and only report the most interesting results.

TRANSPARENCY AND REPRODUCIBILITY

Scientific standards require that AI analyses be reproducible, and AI's complexity makes achieving reproducibility both more critical and more challenging than with traditional methods. Sharing code allows for verification and replication. Making data available (while respecting privacy constraints) enables extension and further testing. Complete documentation of methods, including preprocessing choices, hyperparameters, random seeds, software versions, and implementation details that can influence results, supports meaningful reproduction rather than superficial replication. Thorough reporting of results, including negative findings, uncertainty estimates, robustness checks, and subgroup analyses, promotes honest scientific evaluation. Additionally, preregistering analytical plans prevents the temptation to engage in selective reporting, which AI's exploratory capabilities can foster: when an algorithm can test thousands of model configurations, sharing only the ones that "worked" amounts to a form of analytical misconduct that preregistration helps prevent.

PRIVACY IN ANALYSIS

AI's analytical power introduces privacy risks that traditional methods did not pose. Advanced pattern recognition can enable reidentification of individuals from supposedly deidentified datasets through linkage, inference, or exploiting data sparsity. Inference attacks, in which AI deduces sensitive attributes (such as diagnosis, genetic risk, or sexual orientation) not directly measured but implied by measured variables, raise privacy concerns that deidentification of those variables does not resolve. Model memorization, where AI models retain and can reveal specific training examples through adversarial queries, can potentially leak private information even when raw data is not shared.

Privacy-preserving analytical methods reduce these risks. Differential privacy, federated analysis, and synthetic data approaches, discussed in Chapter 13, each involve privacy-utility tradeoffs that researchers must intentionally balance rather than default to either extreme.

DUAL USE AND MISUSE

Analytical capabilities developed for legitimate research can also be used harmfully. Techniques for understanding behavioral patterns might enable manipulation. Predictive models could be repurposed for discriminatory screening. Surveillance methods may be adapted from public health monitoring. Some analytical tools might have military or hostile uses. These dual-use concerns do not preclude the development of analytical methods but highlight the need for responsible disclosure, use restrictions where appropriate, ethical review of potential applications, and ongoing oversight of how research tools are deployed beyond their original purpose.

PRACTICAL IMPLEMENTATION

Organizations implementing AI analysis gain from structured methods that develop capabilities gradually while ensuring quality.

BUILDING ANALYTICAL CAPABILITY

Building institutional AI analytical capacity follows the workforce and infrastructure principles discussed in Chapters 9 and 12, with particular emphasis on methodological support, statisticians, data scientists, and AI specialists who can advise on appropriate methods and prevent misapplication that occurs when researchers adopt tools without understanding their assumptions and limitations.

QUALITY ASSURANCE AND VALIDATION GOVERNANCE

The quality management principles outlined in Chapter 9 require implementation tailored to specific analyses. A methodological review of AI analyses by statisticians or AI specialists who are independent of the analytical team helps identify errors and overlooked assumptions. Reporting checklists, TRIPOD+AI for prediction models and TRIPOD-LLM for large language model studies, ensure comprehensive and standardized reporting.[11,12]

Validation governance should include predefined validation protocols, a clear separation between model development and validation processes (such as different teams or data sources), careful management of validation data to prevent leakage, standardized validation reporting, and continuous performance monitoring of deployed models. These governance structures establish institutional accountability for analytical quality, which individual researcher motivation alone cannot maintain.

INTEGRATION WITH RESEARCH WORKFLOWS

AI analysis works best when integrated into research workflows rather than added after data collection. Engaging analytical experts early in study design enhances both the design and subsequent analysis. Iterative analytical processes, where initial findings guide refinements and validation uncovers issues needing attention, yield more reliable results than one-time analysis. Ongoing documentation of analytical decisions prevents reconstruction problems that occur when months pass between analysis and manuscript preparation. Version control for code and analysis pipelines ensures reproducibility and facilitates collaboration. Additionally, pipeline automation reduces manual errors and undocumented decisions that can undermine reproducibility in complex analytical workflows.

LOOKING FORWARD

AI analytical capabilities keep improving in different directions with direct effects on research.

Foundation models for science, which are large pretrained models adapted for specific research areas, are emerging as powerful tools that offer analytical capabilities with less domain-specific training than purpose-built models need. These models, trained on extensive collections of scientific text, molecular structures, protein sequences, or clinical data, identify domain-specific patterns that can be fine-tuned for particular research questions using relatively small amounts of additional data.

Automated ML (AutoML), which increasingly automates method selection, hyperparameter tuning, and pipeline construction, is democratizing AI analysis by lowering the technical skills needed for implementation. This democratization offers both opportunity (making AI analysis accessible to more researchers) and risk (allowing applications without the necessary methodological understanding to critically evaluate results).

Causal ML, which combines causal inference frameworks with the flexibility of ML, is improving the ability to draw causal conclusions from observational data. This helps bridge the gap between AI's predictive capabilities and the causal understanding that science ultimately aims for. Federated analysis, which processes distributed data without the need for centralization, allows research on sensitive data that could not previously be pooled. Additionally, real-time analytical systems enable adaptive research designs that modify themselves based on the data that accumulates.

Reporting standards continue to evolve. Extensions of CONSORT (for randomized trials), STROBE (for observational studies), and TRIPOD (for prediction models) address AI-specific analytical reporting needs.[11] Fairness standards for assessing and reporting algorithmic bias are developing further. Additionally, reproducibility standards for computational research are establishing clearer expectations for required documentation and sharing.

The trajectory is clear: AI will become essential to scientific analysis in nearly all research fields. The researchers and institutions best suited to advance knowledge will be those that develop true expertise in AI analysis, not just technical skills but also critical evaluation, applying it with thorough validation and interpretation, and retaining the vital human judgment that turns analytical results into scientific understanding.

CONCLUSION

AI is transforming research data analysis, offering capabilities that go far beyond traditional statistical methods. From exploratory analysis and pattern discovery to predictive modeling, causal inference, and multimodal integration, AI allows insights from data at scales and complexities previously impossible.

Foundational frameworks guide responsible use. FUTURE-AI's robustness principle requires analyses to perform reliably under different conditions and resist disruptions.[1] GMLP validation standards call for independent, representative validation with suitable reference standards and continuous monitoring.[2] The NIST Measure function provides comprehensive, context-aware performance assessment.[3] And reporting standards, TRIPOD+AI for prediction models and TRIPOD-LLM for large language model studies, set transparency benchmarks that allow scientific evaluation of AI-assisted results.[11,12]

AI's analytical capabilities come with associated risks. False discoveries, overfitting, algorithmic bias, privacy breaches, and reproducibility issues are ongoing concerns that require careful mitigation through validation, sensitivity analysis, fairness checks, and transparent reporting. Human judgment remains vital and irreplaceable for defining problems, choosing methods, interpreting results, evaluating ethics, and applying context to turn analytical findings into scientific knowledge.

With data analyzed and findings in hand, researchers face important next steps: ensuring research integrity, sharing results, managing peer review, and turning discoveries into impact. These topics, along with training, infrastructure, ethics, and future directions, are covered in the companion volume, *AI for Biomedical Research Volume 2: Quality, Impact, and Implementation.*

KEY TAKEAWAYS

- AI enables analysis of high-dimensional, complex, multimodal data at scales impossible for traditional methods, but powerful tools amplify both genuine findings and spurious patterns.

- FUTURE-AI robustness requires that AI analyses perform reliably under varying conditions, resist perturbations, and maintain temporal stability. Findings that survive only one analytical specification are artifacts, not discoveries.
- GMLP validation emphasizes independent verification on representative data with proper reference standards and continuous monitoring. Validation is a process, not a one-time event.
- Predictive modeling demands thorough validation (cross-validation, external validation, subgroup analysis, and calibration assessment) and careful management of overfitting.
- Deep learning allows advanced analysis of images, text, and multimodal data, achieving landmark results in medical imaging, NLP, and cross-modal prediction.
- Interpretability is vital for scientific validity; inherently interpretable models should be prioritized when performance is comparable, and post hoc explanations must also be validated for accuracy.
- Causal inference with AI demands proper methods and transparent reporting of untestable assumptions that can't be verified from data alone.
- Uncertainty quantification using Bayesian methods, bootstrapping, or conformal prediction offers reliable measures of analytical confidence.
- TRIPOD+AI (2024) and TRIPOD-LLM (2025) set new reporting standards for AI prediction models, replacing the original TRIPOD 2015.
- Ethical considerations encompass algorithmic bias, transparency, privacy (such as reidentification, inference attacks, and model memorization), and dual-use issues.
- Human judgment continues to be crucial for defining problems, choosing methods, interpreting results, evaluating ethics, and the contextual reasoning that turns data into knowledge.

QUESTIONS FOR REFLECTION

1. How could AI analytical skills improve research in your field, and what validation steps are necessary to trust AI-discovered patterns?
2. What interpretability requirements should apply to AI analyses in your research context, and how would you balance interpretability with predictive performance?
3. How can researchers evaluate the robustness of AI analyses, in line with FUTURE-AI principles, given limited resources for extensive testing?
4. What are the biggest risks of AI analysis in your field, such as false findings, algorithmic bias, reproducibility issues, or others, and how can they be addressed?
5. How can your institution develop AI analytical capabilities while ensuring proper quality assurance and human oversight?
6. Which reporting standards (TRIPOD+AI, TRIPOD-LLM, or domain-specific extensions) apply to your research, and how would following them alter your current reporting practices?

NOTES

1. Lekadir, K., et al. (2025). FUTURE-AI: International consensus guideline for trustworthy and deployable artificial intelligence in healthcare. *BMJ*, 388, e081554. https://doi.org/10.1136/bmj-2024-081554. Note: International consensus identifying six core principles, Fairness, Universality, Traceability, Usability, Robustness, and Explainability. The robustness principle, particularly relevant for research analytics, demands reliable performance under varying conditions, resistance to perturbations, graceful degradation, and temporal stability.
2. International Medical Device Regulators Forum. (2025). Good machine learning practice for medical device development: guiding principles. IMDRF/AIML WG/N88 FINAL:2025. https://www.fda.gov/medical-devices/software-medical-device-samd/good-machine-learning-practice-medical-device-development-guiding-principles. Note: Ten guiding principles finalized by IMDRF in January 2025, building on the original 2021 joint

statement by the FDA, Health Canada, and UK MHRA with broader international endorsement and updates including expanded considerations for generative AI, enhanced lifecycle monitoring, and updated data representation requirements. Principles 2 (robust software engineering), 3 (representative datasets), 5 (fit-for-purpose reference standards), and 10 (postdeployment monitoring) are particularly relevant to research data management, establishing that data quality is foundational to trustworthy AI.

3. National Institute of Standards and Technology. (2023). Artificial intelligence risk management framework (AI RMF 1.0). NIST AI 100-1. https://www.nist.gov/itl/ai-risk-management-framework. Note: The Measure function provides structured guidance for comprehensive performance assessment, quantitative metrics, qualitative trustworthiness evaluation, contextual assessment, uncertainty quantification, and comparative benchmarking.
4. McInnes, L., Healy, J., & Melville, J. (2018). UMAP: Uniform manifold approximation and projection for dimension reduction. *arXiv preprint* arXiv:1802.03426. https://arxiv.org/abs/1802.03426. Note: UMAP has become one of the most widely used dimensionality reduction techniques for visualization and exploratory analysis of high-dimensional data, offering computational advantages over t-SNE while preserving both local and global structure.
5. Tibshirani, R. (1996). Regression shrinkage and selection via the lasso. *Journal of the Royal Statistical Society: Series B*, 58(1), 267–288. https://doi.org/10.1111/j.2517-6161.1996.tb02080.x. Note: The foundational paper introducing L1-penalized regression (LASSO), which enables simultaneous variable selection and estimation in high-dimensional settings. Remains one of the most widely used tools in high-dimensional statistics three decades after publication.
6. Robert, C. P., & Casella, G. (2004). *Monte Carlo Statistical Methods*. Springer.
7. Blei, D. M., Kucukelbir, A., & McAuliffe, J. D. (2017). Variational inference: A review for statisticians. *Journal of the American Statistical Association*, 112(518), 859–877. https://doi.org/10.48550/arXiv.1601.00670
8. Gelman, A., Carlin, J. B., Stern, H. S., Dunson, D. B., Vehtari, A., & Rubin, D. B. (2013). *Bayesian Data Analysis* (3rd ed.). Chapman & Hall/CRC. https://doi.org/10.1201/b16018
9. Benjamini, Y., & Hochberg, Y. (1995). Controlling the false discovery rate: A practical and powerful approach to multiple testing. *Journal of the Royal Statistical Society: Series B (Methodological)*, 57(1), 289–300. https://doi.org/10.1111/j.2517-6161.1995.tb02031.x

10. Storey, J. D. (2002). A direct approach to false discovery rates. *Journal of the Royal Statistical Society: Series B (Statistical Methodology)*, 64(3), 479–498.
11. Stephens, M. (2017). False discovery rates: A new deal. *Biostatistics*, 18(2), 275–294. https://doi.org/10.1093/biostatistics/kxw041
12. Barber, R. F., & Candès, E. J. (2015). Controlling the false discovery rate via knockoffs. *The Annals of Statistics*, 43(5), 2055–2085.
13. Benjamini, Y., & Heller, R. (2007). False discovery rates for spatial signals. *Journal of the American Statistical Association*, 102(480), 1272–1281.
14. Efron, B., & Tibshirani, R. J. (1993). *An Introduction to the Bootstrap*. CRC Press. https://doi.org/10.1201/9780429246593
15. Van Calster, B., et al. (2019). Calibration: The achilles heel of predictive analytics. *BMC Medicine*, 17, 230. https://doi.org/10.1186/s12916-019-1466-7
16. Esteva, A., Kuprel, B., Novoa, R. A., Ko, J., Swetter, S. M., Blau, H. M., & Thrun, S. (2017). Dermatologist-level classification of skin cancer with deep neural networks. *Nature*, 542(7639), 115–118. https://doi.org/10.1038/nature21056. Note: Landmark demonstration that a deep CNN trained on ~130,000 clinical images could classify skin cancer at dermatologist-level performance, establishing that deep learning could match expert visual diagnosis in complex medical imaging tasks.
17. Wang, L. L., & Lo, K. (2021). Text mining approaches for dealing with the rapidly expanding literature on COVID-19. *Briefings in Bioinformatics*, 22(2), 781–799. https://doi.org/10.1093/bib/bbaa296. Note: Demonstrates AI text mining at the scale of rapidly accumulating scientific literature, a capability increasingly essential as publication volumes exceed any individual's capacity for manual review.
18. Gallifant, J., et al. (2025). The TRIPOD-LLM reporting guideline for studies using large language models. *Nature Medicine*, 31(1), 60–69. https://doi.org/10.1038/s41591-024-03425-5. Note: Published January 2025, provides specific guidance for transparent reporting of studies using LLMs for prediction, addressing unique LLM characteristics including sensitivity to prompt engineering, potential for training data memorization, and validation challenges when models may have been exposed to evaluation data. As LLMs become embedded in research analytics, this guideline establishes the minimum transparency standard.

19. Lundberg, S. M., & Lee, S. I. (2017). A unified approach to interpreting model predictions. *Advances in Neural Information Processing Systems*, 30, 4765–4774. Note: Introduced SHAP (SHapley Additive exPlanations), which unifies several feature attribution methods under a game-theoretic framework. SHAP values have become the de facto standard for explaining individual predictions from complex machine learning models.
20. Kim, B., et al. (2018). Interpretability beyond feature attribution: Quantitative testing with concept activation vectors (TCAV). *International Conference on Machine Learning.* PMLR, 2018, Stockholm, Sweden.
21. Spirtes, P., Glymour, C., & Scheines, R. (2000). *Causation, Prediction, and Search* (2nd ed.). MIT Press. Note: The foundational text on constraint-based causal discovery algorithms (PC, FCI), establishing the theoretical framework for inferring causal structure from conditional independence patterns in observational data.
22. Kaufman, S., Rosset, S., Perlich, C., & Stitelman, O. (2012). Leakage in data mining: Formulation, detection, and avoidance. ACM Transactions on Knowledge Discovery from Data, 6(4), 15, 21. https://doi.org/10.1145/2382577.2382579
23. Vovk, V., Gammerman, A., & Shafer, G. (2005). *Algorithmic Learning in a Random World.* Springer. Note: The foundational text on conformal prediction, a distribution-free framework providing prediction intervals with guaranteed finite-sample coverage under minimal assumptions. Conformal prediction has gained substantial momentum in AI research since 2020 as a practical approach to uncertainty quantification that works with any underlying model.
24. Collins, G. S., Moons, K. G. M., Dhiman, P., Riley, R. D., Beam, A. L., Van Calster, B., & Snell, K. I. E. (2024). TRIPOD+AI statement: Updated guidance for reporting clinical prediction models that use regression or machine learning methods. *BMJ*, 385, e078378. https://doi.org/10.1136/bmj-2023-078378. Note: This 27-item checklist supersedes the original TRIPOD 2015 statement. TRIPOD+AI provides harmonized guidance for reporting prediction model studies regardless of whether regression or machine learning methods are used, addressing AI-specific reporting needs including model architecture, training procedures, and comprehensive validation characterization.

Epilogue
From Analysis to Impact

THE JOURNEY SO FAR

This book has traced the transformation of research through artificial intelligence (AI) across every stage of the research lifecycle. The initial chapters examined how AI reshapes the intellectual foundations of research, helping researchers identify promising questions, synthesize extensive literatures, generate hypotheses, and design rigorous studies. AI then expands into the organizational aspects of research, writing competitive grant proposals, assembling effective teams, optimizing research portfolios, and managing the administrative and compliance tasks that take up so much researcher time. Throughout these chapters, AI consistently acts as a force multiplier for human ability rather than a replacement.

The later chapters focus on the core operational and analytical aspects of research execution. Governance frameworks, RUAIH, FUTURE-AI, NIST AI RMF, and GMLP, were developed within the context of institutional review board and ethics review and then implemented across various areas such as participant recruitment, research operations, data collection and management, and data analysis and interpretation. Each application domain presented unique challenges: balancing efficiency with fairness in recruitment, supporting team well-being while optimizing operations, ensuring data quality and traceability at large scales, and maintaining scientific rigor when AI's analytical capabilities make it easy to detect patterns everywhere. The regulatory landscape, from ICH E6(R3) to the EU AI Act and emerging FDA guidance, is rapidly shaping the governance infrastructure for AI-enhanced research.

Across all 14 chapters, several constants surfaced: AI's exceptional capabilities must be complemented by thorough validation, transparency fosters the trust needed for scientific progress, equity requires active effort rather than passive hope, and human judgment, in framing questions, analyzing results, and making ethical choices, remains essential. These principles guide each chapter's discussion and lay the groundwork for what follows.

WHAT ANALYSIS REVEALS AND WHAT REMAINS

Reaching the analysis stage represents a significant milestone. Data have been collected according to carefully designed protocols. Quality has been assured. Patterns have been identified, models built, and hypotheses tested. The researcher now has findings, results that may confirm or challenge expectations, answer questions or raise new ones, advance understanding, or reveal how much remains unknown.

But analysis is not the end of research. It is, in many ways, a beginning.

Findings must be validated, not just through the internal validation procedures discussed in Chapter 14 but through the broader processes of scientific scrutiny that determine whether results are genuine, reproducible, and meaningful. Research integrity requires vigilance against error, bias, and misconduct, with AI offering both new tools for detecting problems and new challenges as AI-generated content becomes more prevalent.

Results must be communicated, first to scientific peers through publications and presentations and then to broader audiences including practitioners, policymakers, and the public. Effective science communication has always required skill; AI is transforming both the tools available for communication and the landscape into which scientific findings are disseminated.

Publications must survive peer review, a system under strain from increasing submission volumes, reproducibility concerns, and now questions about AI-generated content and AI-assisted review. Understanding how AI is changing peer review is essential for researchers navigating this evolving system.

Research must achieve impact and be translated into practice, policy, products, or further investigation. The gap between discovery and application has long concerned research stakeholders; AI offers new opportunities to accelerate translation while raising questions about responsible deployment.

The research enterprise itself must be sustained, through training new researchers, maintaining infrastructure, managing resources, and adapting to technological change. Institutions must implement AI capabilities thoughtfully, managing change while building capacity for an AI-enhanced future.

And throughout, ethical, legal, and social implications demand attention. The governance frameworks introduced in this book, RUAIH, FUTURE-AI, NIST AI RMF, GMLP, and the EU AI Act, represent emerging consensus on responsible AI use, but their implementation requires ongoing attention and adaptation as AI capabilities and applications evolve. The foundational ethical principles established in Chapter 1, transparency, accountability, fairness, privacy, beneficence, scientific integrity, and respect for human agency, grounded in the Belmont Report's enduring principles of respect for persons, beneficence, and justice and extended by NIST's Belmont-AI initiative, provide the moral foundation within which all governance frameworks operate.

THE COMPANION VOLUME

These crucial topics, everything that happens after analysis, are the subject of the companion volume, *AI for Biomedical Research Volume 2: Quality, Impact, and Implementation.* That book continues the journey with:

Research Integrity and Quality explores how AI both challenges and supports scientific integrity, from detecting fabrication and plagiarism to ensuring reproducibility in today's complex computational analyses.

Dissemination and Communication examines AI tools for scientific writing, visualization, and public engagement, while also addressing concerns about AI-generated misinformation and the evolving information landscape.

Peer Review and Publication examines how AI is transforming scholarly publishing, from AI-assisted review to preprint servers and new models of scientific communication.

Research Impact and Translation explores how AI can speed up the move from discovery to application, while making sure that translation is responsible and fair.

Training and Education examines how AI is transforming research training, from AI-enhanced curricula to new skills researchers must acquire in an AI-enabled environment.

Infrastructure and Resource Management covers the computational, data, and human infrastructure needed for AI-driven research, including sustainability and equity factors.

Ethical, Legal, and Social Implications provide a comprehensive examination of AI governance frameworks, comparing voluntary and mandatory approaches and exploring emerging ethical challenges.

Implementation and Change Management provides practical guidance for institutions adopting AI capabilities, focusing on organizational change, workforce development, and sustainable implementation.

Future Directions considers emerging AI capabilities, changing regulatory landscapes, and the long-term path of AI in research.

Together, the two volumes offer comprehensive coverage of AI throughout the entire research cycle, from the initial spark of an idea to lasting impact and the sustainable infrastructure necessary to keep advancing knowledge.

PRINCIPLES FOR THE AI-ENHANCED RESEARCHER

The principles guiding researchers engaging with AI are woven throughout this book rather than saved for a final summary. They start with the ethical foundations from Chapter 1, including transparency, accountability, fairness, privacy, beneficence, scientific integrity, and respect for human agency, and become more specific through the governance frameworks discussed in Chapters 2–14. Readers revisiting this epilogue for a quick review will find the most detailed coverage of ethical principles in Chapter 1, governance frameworks in Chapter 9, and evaluating AI products in Chapter 10. These principles remain constant; their applications will continue to adapt.

LOOKING FORWARD

We are at a historic moment in research. AI provides capabilities that once seemed like science fiction a generation ago, such as reading and synthesizing thousands of papers, analyzing complex datasets using advanced methods, generating human-quality text and images, and serving as intellectual partners in research.

These capabilities present both opportunities and responsibilities. The opportunity lies in accelerating discovery, solving problems once considered impossible, democratizing access to advanced analytical tools, and reducing administrative tasks that have long distracted researchers from science itself. The responsibility involves using these capabilities wisely, ensuring proper validation, ethical consideration, attention to fairness, and preserving the human judgment that gives research its purpose and guidance.

This book aims to offer practical guidance for seizing opportunities while fulfilling responsibilities. The chapters cover specific applications, identify relevant frameworks, acknowledge limitations, and present implementation strategies. However, no book can provide all the answers for a technology that evolves as quickly as AI.

What this book offers, and what I hope it has offered, is a foundation for thinking about AI in research: understanding what AI can and cannot do (right now), knowing which frameworks guide responsible use, recognizing both capabilities and limitations, and valuing the ongoing importance of human judgment in the research process.

The companion volume continues this exploration, focusing on what happens after analysis and how institutions can develop sustainable AI capabilities. Together, the two volumes aim to prepare researchers, administrators, and research institutions for an AI-driven future.

The transformation of research through AI has only just begun. The researchers who will guide that change, use AI responsibly, oppose its misuse, and protect what matters most in scientific inquiry are reading these words now.

The work continues.

Index

Note: **Bold** page numbers refer to tables.

C

E

J

K

L

M

N

O

S

T

U

V

W

For Product Safety Concerns and Information please contact our EU
representative GPSR@taylorandfrancis.com
Taylor & Francis Verlag GmbH, Kaufingerstraße 24, 80331 München, Germany

www.ingramcontent.com/pod-product-compliance
Lightning Source LLC
La Vergne TN
LVHW010738171026
850310LV00031B/204

* 9 7 8 1 0 4 1 3 2 3 3 9 6 *